PUBLIC HEALTH IN THE

CHILD EXPOSURE TO ELEMENTAL MERCURY

PUBLIC HEALTH IN THE 21ST CENTURY

Additional books in this series can be found on Nova's website under the Series tab.

Additional E-books in this series can be found on Nova's website under the E-books tab.

PUBLIC HEALTH IN THE 21ST CENTURY

CHILD EXPOSURE TO ELEMENTAL MERCURY

RIITTA A. RUSTOEN
AND
SERENA R. ZIEGLER
EDITORS

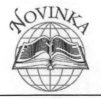

Nova Science Publishers, Inc.
New York

Library of Congress Cataloging-in-Publication Data

ISBN 978-1-61470-941-1

Published by Nova Science Publishers, Inc. † New York

CONTENTS

PREFACE

Mercury occurs naturally in the environment and exists in several forms. Elemental mercury, also known as metallic of liquid mercury, is a unique metal that forms a dense, silvery liquid at room temperature. The liquid can disperse and coalesces into small, shiny droplets. These unusual properties attract the interest of children, increasing their propensity to play with mercury. Mercury vapor is readily absorbed by the lungs, making inhalation of elemental mercury the exposure route of greatest concern. The health effects that may result from mercury vary with the magnitude, dose, and duration of exposure. This book examines and identifies the common sources of elemental mercury exposure in children and describes the location, demographics, and proportion of children exposed or potentially exposed to elemental mercury in the United States.

Chapter 1- In Franklinville, New Jersey, an industrial building formerly used to manufacture mercury thermometers was renovated and converted in 2004 to a children's daycare facility. Unfortunately, the renovated property was not cleaned up prior to renovation, leaving residual contamination with elemental mercury. Such contamination can cause significant exposure to children or adults who are present. In these types of exposure events the persons exposed may require medical evaluation and biomonitoring. Congress directed the Agency for Toxic Substances and Disease Registry (ATSDR) to further investigate and characterize these exposures.

Chapter 2- Mercury is an element and a metal that is found in air, water, and soil. It exists in three forms that have different properties, usage, and toxicity. The three forms are called elemental (or metallic) mercury, inorganic mercury compounds, and organic mercury compounds.

In: Child Exposure to Elemental Mercury   ISBN: 978-1-61470-941-1
Editors: R. Rustoen and S. Ziegler   © 2012 Nova Science Publishers, Inc.

Chapter 1

CHILDREN'S EXPOSURE TO ELEMENTAL MERCURY: A NATIONAL REVIEW OF EXPOSURE EVENTS*

Centers for Disease Control and Prevention

ABBREVIATIONS, ACRONYMS, TERMINOLOGY

%	Percent
≤	Less than or equal to
<	Less than
AAPCC	American Association of Poison Control Centers
ATSDR	Agency for Toxic Substances and Disease Registry
°C	Celsius
CDC	Centers for Disease Control and Prevention
CERCLA	Comprehensive Environmental Response, Compensation, and Liability Act (aka Superfund)
CI	Confidence Interval
CFL	Compact Florescent Lightbulb
EPA	U.S. Environmental Protection Agency
g/cm^3	Grams per Cubic Centimeter
g	Grams

---

* This is an edited, reformatted and augmented version of a Centers for Disease Control and Prevention publication, dated February 2009.

HC	Health Consultation
HSEES	Hazardous Substances Emergency Events Surveillance
IDPH	Illinois Department of Public Health
LOD	Level of Detection
MDCH	Michigan Department of Community Health
ml	Milliliter
mm	Millimeter
n	Number
NHANES	National Health and Nutrition Examination Survey
NIOSH	National Institute for Occupational Safety and Health
NPL	National Priorities List (lists the 1,300 most polluted hazardous waste sites)
NRC	National Response Center
PEHSU	Pediatric Environmental Health Specialty Units
$\mu g/g$	Micrograms per gram
$\mu g/L$	Micrograms per Liter
$\mu g/m^3$	Micrograms per Cubic Meter

1. EXECUTIVE SUMMARY

1.1. Introduction

In Franklinville, New Jersey, an industrial building formerly used to manufacture mercury thermometers was renovated and converted in 2004 to a children's daycare facility [ATSDR 2007b]. Unfortunately, the renovated property was not cleaned up prior to renovation, leaving residual contamination with elemental mercury [ATSDR 2007b]. Such contamination can cause significant exposure to children or adults who are present. In these types of exposure events the persons exposed may require medical evaluation and biomonitoring. Congress directed the Agency for Toxic Substances and Disease Registry (ATSDR) to further investigate and characterize these exposures.

The Explanatory Statement to the Fiscal Year (FY) 2008 Appropriation for the Agency for Toxic Substances and Disease Registry stated the following:

From within the amount appropriated, ATSDR is expected to assess the extent of children's exposure to mercury from former industrial sites and other sources nationwide, and to issue a report of its findings 12 months after the date of enactment of this bill. (Consolidated Appropriations Act, 2008 Committee Print of the House Committee on Appropriations on H.R. 2764/Public Law 110-1 61, page 1278).

This article was prepared by ATSDR in response to this request.

1.2. Background

Mercury occurs naturally in the environment and exists in several forms. Between 0.006 and 0.02 µg/m^3 have been reported in outdoor air [ATSDR 1999]. Elemental mercury, also known as metallic or liquid mercury, is a unique metal that forms a dense, silvery liquid at room temperature. The liquid can disperse and coalesces into small, shiny droplets. These unusual properties attract the interest of children, increasing their propensity to play with mercury [Azziz-Baumgartner et al. 2007; Lowry et al. 1999].

Liquid mercury has a relatively low vapor pressure (0.0085 mm mercury at 25°C) and volatilizes slowly at room temperature. Mercury vapor is readily absorbed by the lungs, making inhalation of elemental mercury the exposure route of greatest concern. The health effects that may result from mercury exposure vary with the magnitude, dose, and duration of exposure.

1.3. Objective

To address the Congressional directive, ATSDR in collaboration with the Centers for Disease Control and Prevention (CDC), formed the ATSDR\CDC Mercury Workgroup. The objectives of the workgroup were to:

1) identify the common sources of elemental mercury exposure in children; and
2) describe the location, demographics, and proportion of children exposed or potentially exposed to elemental mercury in the United States.

In this document, elemental mercury refers to metallic mercury, a silvery liquid that vaporizes slowly at room temperature. Specifically excluded from this report are mercury exposures from coal-burning facilities, dental amalgams, fish consumption, medical waste incinerators, and vaccines. These exclusions are necessary to focus the report on the elemental mercury exposure events that formed the impetus for the Congressional directive.

1.4. Methods

Information was sought on mercury-related events that were documented to expose (or potentially expose) children in the United States. A comprehensive review of these events was conducted to identify and quantify the most common and recent exposure sources and to describe the location, demographics, and proportion of children affected.

The data sources reviewed included an extensive list of federal, state, and regional programs that capture information on spills and other hazardous releases. Once the events were selected, the characteristics of each event (i.e., the source, location, and demographics of the children affected) were explored.

The various databases that contain information about specific childhood mercury exposures often contain relatively few details. To supplement the information from these data sources, a search of the published scientific literature was also conducted.

The Mercury Workgroup also reviewed a number of prevention initiatives and information resources for reducing mercury exposure. This information is provided in the Appendix as supplemental material.

1.5. Findings

Public health databases were reviewed for relevant information on elemental mercury-related exposure events. The information presented is from the five relevant sources: 1) ATSDR - Health Consultations and Emergency Response Calls, 2) ATSDR - Hazardous Substances Emergency Events Surveillance (HSEES), 3) U.S. Coast Guard - National Response Center (NRC) database, 4) American Association of Poison Control Centers (AAPCC) - National Poison Data System, and 5) Association of Occupational and Environmental Clinics (AOEC) - Pediatric Environmental Health Specialty Units (PEHSU).

A TSDR - Health Consultations and Emergency Response Calls. During 2002 to 2007, 26 health consultations were produced for events that exposed or potentially exposed children to elemental mercury in air. Although not always mutually exclusive, the location of the exposure event was most frequently described as a home (46%; 12 of 26) or school (42%; 11 of 26). The source of these mercury exposures included mercury use or storage in schools, mercury release from broken thermometers or sphygmomanometers, off-gassing from flooring containing a mercury catalyst, and an unknown source.

ATSDR - Hazardous Substances Emergency Events Surveillance. From 2002 through 2006, there were 843 mercury related events, 409 were classified as potentially exposing children. Mercury events occurred most frequently in private households (75%; 307 of 409). The most frequent contributing cause of the event was human error (87%; 357 of 409). The human error category includes breaking of or dropping thermometers or other mercury-containing devices or equipment. The total number of people exposed was not captured, although 21 people (10 children) reported injuries or symptoms.

U.S. Coast Guard - National Response Center Database. The National Response Center receives between 25,000 and 30,000 reports of pollution incidents and response drills each year. Of the mercury incidents reported between 2002 and 2007, 113 were events in which children were potentially exposed. The amount of mercury released varied from less than 1 ml to approximately 1,893 ml.

AAPCC - National Poison Data System. Between 2002 and 2006, there were 6,396 calls made to Poison Control Centers regarding children's exposure to elemental mercury not associated with broken thermometers. During the same time periods there were 30,891 calls made to Poison Control Centers regarding children's exposure to mercury from broken thermometers. From 2002 to 2006, the calls for children exposed to mercury thermometers have decreased from 10,108 to 2,896. Most non- thermometer (93%; 5,966 of 6,396) and thermometer-related (98%; 30,287 of 30,891) calls were classified as being minimal to nontoxic in nature.

AOEC - *Pediatric Environmental Health Specialty Unit.* Between 2004 and 2007, 242 mercury exposure calls were made; 120 (50%) concerned potentially exposed boys, 93 (3 8%) concerned girls, and the sex of the remaining 29 (12%) was not identified. The majority of these calls concerned children less than 7 years old.

Literature Review. Ten published reports, described 13 mercury contamination events with approximately 1,393 exposed children between 1998 and 2004. When reported, the estimated amount of mercury spilled/released ranged from 9 to 701 ml. The largest releases typically occurred after children stole mercury from an industrial site (approximately 701 ml mercury released) or a school (30–40 ml mercury released). In eight events a child obtained mercury by stealing. Mercury was stolen from a school in 6 of the 13 events (46%), once from a dental office (8%), and once from an industrial site (8%). When biologic specimens were collected to assess human exposure to mercury neither urine nor blood mercury levels correlated well with the presence or severity of symptoms [Cherry et al. 2002; Gattineni et al. 2007; Tominack et al. 2002].

1.6. Discussion and Conclusions

Review of the data sources and literature found three categories of exposure scenarios. The first two categories are scenarios in the home and those at school, two common locations for childhood elemental mercury exposures. The third category includes exposures at other locations, such as medical clinics and property that was not adequately remediated. The sources of exposure in the home include mercury- containing devices, cultural or ceremonial uses of mercury, intentionally heating elemental mercury, and unknowingly tracking mercury home from the workplace. The most common elemental mercury sources in schools are mercury stored in science laboratories, mercury found in broken instruments, and mercury brought to school from other locations. In addition, some gymnasium floors contain a mercury catalyst that can release mercury vapor into the air. Mercury exposures can also occur in medical facilities and buildings where mercury was previously used. Sources include prior mercury spills, mercury stored on abandoned property, and mercury found in medical or dental offices. In some cases, mercury is carried or tracked into multiple locations, making it difficult to identify the primary location where exposure first took place.

Regardless of exposure location, children are most frequently exposed to mercury when mercury is mishandled or when people improperly clean up spilled mercury. Exposure to small spills from broken thermometers represents the most frequent scenario. However, calls about this type of exposure are decreasing. Elevated mercury vapor levels have been documented, but demonstrable health effects are rarely reported after small mercury spills such as broken fever thermometers. Regardless, proper clean up of even small spills should occur.

Limitations. The demographics and proportion of U.S. children exposed is not directly quantifiable using the various data sources reviewed. Most data sources that collect information on the release of hazardous substances do not systematically collect information on the persons affected. Furthermore, the duplication and inconsistent reporting of the events between data sources and even within data sources make any estimate of the national incidence of mercury exposure to children unreliable.

Examples and Resources for Reducing Mercury Exposure. The review of prevention initiatives and information resources found that a number of federal and state-based initiatives affect the potential for childhood mercury exposures. Currently, there are 45 states with mercury initiatives. The supplemental material in the Appendix describes ongoing federal and state initiatives that are examples of ways to reduce exposure to elemental mercury. Information sources are summarized and are useful to organizations or individuals seeking information on preventing mercury exposures, responding appropriately to environmental contamination, and evaluating and caring for exposed children.

Published case reports and case series often provide exposure and health outcome information but are limited by reporting bias, retrospective data collection, and imprecise estimates of exposure dose and duration. Despite their limitations, the data sources and literature reviewed in this report are the most current and best available data sources on acute exposures to mercury in the United States.

2. INTRODUCTION

2.1. Congressional Directive

In recent years, mercury contamination events have been documented at private residences or daycare centers that were converted from industrial facilities that used mercury. Residual contamination in these locations can result in significant exposure to people who are present and can be costly to clean [Baughman 2006; NJDEP 2008; SHP 2003].

One such event was reported in 2006 in Franklinville, New Jersey [ATSDR 2007b]. A building formerly used to manufacture mercury thermometers was renovated and converted to a daycare facility for children.

Residual elemental mercury contamination on the property resulted in a mercury exposure event. Numerous children who spent time at the daycare required medical evaluation and biomonitoring.

Congress directed the Agency for Toxic Substances and Disease Registry (ATSDR) to further investigate and characterize these exposures. The Explanatory Statement to the Fiscal Year (FY) 2008 Appropriation for the Agency for Toxic Substances and Disease Registry (ATSDR) stated the following:

> *From within the amount appropriated, ATSDR is expected to assess the extent of children's exposure to mercury from former industrial sites and other sources nationwide, and to issue a report of its findings 12 months after the date of enactment of this bill. (Consolidated Appropriations Act, 2008 Committee Print of the House Committee on Appropriations on H.R. 2764/Public Law 110-1 61, page 1278)*

To address the Congressional directive, ATSDR in collaboration with the Centers for Disease Control and Prevention (CDC) formed the ATSDR\CDC Mercury Workgroup.

2.2. Objectives

The objectives of the Mercury Workgroup were to:

1) identify the exposure sources associated with elemental mercury exposure in children; and
2) describe the location, demographics, and proportion of children exposed or potentially exposed to elemental mercury in the United States.

The Mercury Workgroup reported on elemental mercury exposures that typically occur when children inhale mercury vapor related to:

- disposal or damage to mercury devices (e.g., thermometers or lightbulbs);
- off-gassing of mercury vapors from flooring materials;

- proximity to industrial sites or hazardous waste sites contaminated with mercury;
- reuse of industrial property contaminated with mercury;
- residential contamination caused by religious or cultural practices; and
- release of mercury found in school science laboratories or health care facilities.

The Mercury Workgroup did not review mercury exposures associated with coal- burning facilities, dental amalgams, fish consumption, medical waste incinerators, or thimerosal-containing vaccines. Nor did it focus on elemental mercury health effects.

3. BACKGROUND

3.1. Mercury Forms and Properties of Elemental Mercury

Mercury is a naturally occurring element in the earth's crust. It exists in the environment as the result of natural processes and human activities.
The three chemical forms are:

1) elemental mercury (also called liquid or metallic mercury);
2) inorganic mercury compounds, including common compounds formed from the monovalent and divalent cations of mercury (e.g., mercurous chloride, mercuric chloride, mercuric acetate, and mercuric sulfide); and
3) organic mercury compounds, most commonly found in the form of methylmercury or ethylmercury [ATSDR 1999; Clarkson 2002].

Elemental mercury is a unique metal that forms a dense, silvery liquid at room temperature (density = 13.534 g/cm^3). The liquid can disperse and coalesces into small, shiny droplets. These unusual properties attract the interest of children, increasing their propensity to play with mercury [Azziz-Baumgartner et al. 2007; Lowry et al. 1999]. Liquid mercury has a relatively low vapor pressure (0.0085 mm mercury at 25°C) and volatilizes slowly at room temperature. Indoor mercury spills that are not properly cleaned up can release mercury vapors into the air for weeks or even years [ATSDR 1999]. Heating mercury results in much higher, potentially lethal, airborne mercury concentrations, especially in indoor spaces [Putman and Madden 1972; Solis et al. 2000; Taueg et al. 1992].

3.2. Toxicokinetics of Elemental Mercury

Mercury vapor is readily absorbed by the lungs, making inhalation of elemental mercury the exposure route of greatest concern [Hursh et al. 1976].Although children may sometimes swallow elemental mercury, it is poorly absorbed in the normal gastrointestinal tract. In animal studies, less than 0.0 1% of the elemental mercury ingested was absorbed [WHO 1991]. Dermal absorption of elemental mercury is also a relatively minor exposure pathway. When human volunteers were exposed to mercury vapor, the estimated uptake rate through the skin was approximately 2% of the uptake rate through the lungs [Hursh et al. 1989].

After absorption, elemental mercury is distributed to most tissues, with the highest concentrations occurring in the kidney [Barregard et al. 1999; Hursh et al. 1976]. Elemental mercury is mostly oxidized to inorganic forms and excreted by the kidneys [Sandborgh-Englund et al. 1998]. Blood concentrations decline initially during a relatively rapid clearance phase, with a half-life of approximately 1–3 days. This rapid phase is followed by a slower clearance phase, with a half-life of 1–3 weeks [Barregard et al. 1992; Sandborgh-Englund et al. 1998]. Peak urine mercury levels can lag behind peak blood levels by days to a few weeks [Barregard et al. 1992]; thereafter, urinary mercury levels decline with a half-life of 1–3 months [Jonsson et al. 1999; Roels et al. 1991].

3.3. Elemental Mercury Exposure Pathways

Exposure to mercury occurs through a variety of pathways. These exposures result from spills and misuse of mercury in homes, schools, and other locations. Although some mercury-containing devices are becoming less common in the home, mercury is still found in a number of household items including: thermometers, barometers, thermostats, lightbulbs, electric switches, and natural gas regulators. Even the small amount of mercury in a typical thermometer (0.5 to 3.0 g mercury or 0.04 to 0.22 ml mercury) can create hazardous conditions if spilled indoors and improperly cleaned [Smart 1986; von Muhlendahl 1990]. For example, vacuuming can result in additional dispersion of elemental mercury, which increases the inhalational hazard and spreads the contamination. The ATSDR Minimal Risk Levels for chronic mercury inhalation is 0.2 $\mu g/m^3$ [ATSDR 1999].

Some Caribbean religions and folk healers use mercury for religious or ceremonial purposes [Wendroff 2005]. The ceremonial uses of mercury include applying it to the skin, adding it to candles, or sprinkling it around the home. Elemental mercury is easily dispersed into fine beads that sink into carpets, furniture, cracks in the floor, or other porous materials (Figure 1a, 1b). Mercury tracked from room to room produces widespread contamination throughout the house. These practices can potentially expose practitioners and their children. Following indoor spills, mercury can persist for months and even years [Carpi and Chen 2001]. Therefore ceremonial use of mercury in the home could also expose future occupants and their children. Occasionally, mercury contamination is so extensive that adequate cleaning is not possible and the building must be demolished [Orloff et al. 1997].

Reports have indicated that children have been exposed to mercury vapors from polyurethane flooring materials in some schools [ATSDR 2003, 2004]. In addition, school science laboratories may store elemental mercury and various types of mercury-containing equipment, such as thermometers and barometers. Elemental mercury has unique physical properties that attract children. Older children may obtain mercury by scavenging from schools, abandoned buildings, or other locations. Children who take mercury home may play with it and share it with their friends, contaminating other homes.

Especially in the western United States, abandoned mines and precious metal recovery operations are sometimes extensively contaminated with elemental mercury. At such sites, large amounts of elemental mercury mixed in the soil can expose children who venture onto the site [Rytuba 2000].

Although children are not typically exposed to mercury in active workplaces, some former industrial facilities that used mercury are subsequently converted to residences or childcare facilities. Inadequate remediation of such properties can lead to significant exposure [ATSDR 1998, 2007b]. Current work sites can also pose a hazard if workers carry mercury home on their clothes and shoes, exposing other family members [Hudson et al. 1987].

3.4. Biomarkers of Elemental Mercury Exposure

After absorption, elemental mercury is converted to inorganic mercury and excreted in the urine. Therefore, urine levels provide the most appropriate assessment of elemental mercury exposure and are the easiest to interpret [ATSDR 1999]. Serial urine levels are sometimes used to ensure that exposure is not continuing.

The amount of mercury in blood is sometimes measured during the first 3 days after an exposure because blood mercury levels peak sooner than urine levels [ATSDR 1999]. However, the presence of organic mercury from an individual's diet complicates the interpretation of blood mercury levels [Clarkson 2002], and few commercial laboratories differentiate between the various mercury species in blood.

Mercury is also measurable in hair. However, these tests primarily measure organic mercury [Aposhian et al. 1992; ATSDR 2001c; Cianciola et al. 1997; Kingman et al. 1998], and are not useful for assessing recent exposures to elemental mercury.

3.5. Reference Levels in U.S. Children

The CDC's National Center for Health Statistics conducts the National Health and Nutrition Examination Survey (NHANES) to assess the health and nutrition status of the civilian, noninstitutionalized U.S. population. NHANES data provide mercury reference levels in U.S. children and markers of exposure for the general population. NHANES data are representative samples based on a complex multistage probability sampling design [CDC 2007].

Urine mercury levels were measured in participants aged 6 years and older in the 2003–2004 NHANES survey period. For children aged 6 to 11 years, the geometric mean[1] was 0.254 µg/L (95% confidence interval [CI]: 0.2 13–0.304) and 0.358 µg/L (95% CI: 0.313–0.408) for children 12 to 19 years of age [CDC 2005c, 2007]. Table 1 provides additional urine mercury reference levels.

In 2001–2002 NHANES measured blood mercury levels in young children (aged 1–5 years). The geometric mean was 0.32 µg/L (95% CI: 0.27–0.3 8), and the 95th percentile was 1.2 µg/L (95% CI 0.9–1.6) [CDC 2005c].

NHANES urine mercury reference levels are similar to background urinary mercury levels reported in German children [Link et al. 2007].

3.6. Overview on Health Effects of Elemental Mercury Exposure

The health effects that may result from mercury vary with the magnitude, dose, and duration of exposure. Children are more sensitive to mercury and thus at greater risk than adults from certain exposures [ATSDR 1999; Rogers et al. 2007]. Children breathe faster and have larger lung surface areas relative to body weight than adults, resulting in a greater dose of mercury per unit of body weight. Children are shorter in stature than adults and engage in activities such as crawling or playing on the floor. As a result, their breathing zones are closer to the floor, where mercury vapor levels are higher. The types of health effects are further described according to the duration of exposure (acute vs. chronic).

The health effects from inhaling very high concentrations of mercury are primarily respiratory in nature [ATSDR 1999; EPA 2002]. These health effects may include pneumonitis, bronchiolitis, pulmonary edema, and even death [ATSDR 1999; Solis et al. 2000; Taueg et al. 1992].

Exposure to mercury vapor (e.g., 10–100 $\mu g/m^3$) over prolonged time periods can cause neurobehavioral effects, including mood changes and tremors. Chronic exposure can also cause hypertension and autonomic nervous system dysfunction [WHO 2003]. Low urinary mercury levels (e.g., <5 $\mu g/L$ urine) have not been associated with neurocognitive effects in children [Bellinger et al. 2006; DeRouen et al. 2006].

Mercury exposure is also associated with acrodynia (painful extremities), a rare syndrome believed to result from hypersensitivity to mercury [Caravati et al. 2008; von Muhlendahl 1990; Warkany 1966; Wossmann et al. 1999]. Acrodynia is more common among small children, who develop nonspecific symptoms such as leg cramps, irritability, and redness and peeling of skin on the hands, nose, and feet [Tunnessen et al. 1987]. Acrodynia was more common in the past when mercury- containing laxatives, teething powders, and diaper rinses were widely used [Tunnessen et al. 1987].

There is not always a correlation between exposure levels and health effects. In addition, while elevated mercury vapor levels have been documented, demonstrable health effects are rarely reported after small mercury spills such as broken fever thermometers. Additional health effects information is available in the ATSDR Mercury Toxicological Profile [ATSDR 1999] and in the World Health Organization Concise International Chemical Assessment Documents on mercury [WHO 2003].

4. METHODS

Information was sought on mercury-related events that were documented to expose (or potentially expose) children in the United States. A comprehensive review of these events was conducted to identify and quantify the most common and recent exposure sources and to describe the location, demographics, and proportion of children affected.

The Mercury Workgroup also reviewed a number of prevention initiatives and information resources. This information is provided in the Appendix as supplemental materials.

4.1. Data Sources

The data sources reviewed included an extensive list of federal, state, and regional programs that capture information on spills and other hazardous releases. Initially, a list of databases and public health entities that collect mercury-related health and exposure information was compiled (Table 2). Workgroup members then identified and contacted key personnel for each relevant data source.

Many of the data sources depend on individuals to report releases or spills to a regulatory authority. Information about the nature and extent of such releases is limited by the potential implications for remediation and legal liability. The findings section assesses and reports the limitations of each data source ("8. Findings—Data Sources").

4.2. Exposure Event Selection Criteria

Mercury-related events that were documented to expose (or potentially expose) children in the United States were obtained from each data source. The following guidelines were used to select relevant mercury releases and spills (exposure events) for this report.

First, the time period reviewed was generally between 2002 and 2007. Although this time frame represents the most current information available on exposure events, these dates were somewhat flexible to allow for differences in the data sources and completeness of the reported data. In some instances, data from a longer period of time were used to include pertinent events. The actual time period reviewed is reported for each data source.

Second, the event took place in the continental United States, Alaska, Hawaii, or Puerto Rico.

Lastly, the event exposed or potentially affected a child (or children) 18 years of age or younger. Although an attempt was made to query events in which children were 18 years of age or younger, these ages were somewhat flexible to allow for differences in the data sources and completeness of the reported data. If the data source did not contain information on the age of persons exposed or affected, the event location became the determining factor. That is, the event was included if it occurred at a location thought to be frequented by children (e.g., an elementary or secondary school, a daycare, or a private residence).

Once the events were selected, the characteristics of each event (i.e., the source, location, and demographics of the children affected) were explored. The reporting methodology differs among data sources, and the information available also differs in content and definition. In an attempt to obtain reasonably comparable mercury event characteristics, the following information was collected for each event when it was available:

- year and date of event,
- location of event (state, city),
- event location type (e.g., daycare),
- form of mercury released,
- amount of mercury released,
- number of children potentially exposed,
- the ages of affected children,
- estimated length of exposure,
- possible contributing causes of the release/spill,
- recorded mercury vapor levels, and
- blood or urine mercury levels.

The findings section provides a detailed description of the available data by data source ("8. Findings—Data Sources").

4.3. Literature Review

The various databases that contain information about specific childhood mercury exposures often contain relatively few details. To supplement the information from these data sources, a search of the published scientific literature was also conducted.

Literature searches were conducted in PubMed and the Web of Science for published reports of mercury exposures involving children. The searches were limited to exposures that occurred in the United States. The search terms included "elemental mercury," "metallic mercury," or "liquid mercury." Only publications between January 2002 and December 2007 were reviewed. Publications in which urine mercury levels in children were measured without documentation of an exposure event were omitted.

4.4. Presentation of Findings

Findings are presented in three major sections. The first section ("8. Findings—Data Sources") identifies the data sources, describes the data, and summarizes the applicable information. The second section ("9. Findings—Literature Review") includes results from the review of the published, scientific literature. The third section ("10. Findings—Exposure Scenarios") uses the information reported in the first two sections along with additional case reports to characterize typical exposure locations. Specific scenarios are included in this section to illustrate typical exposures at each location.

5. FINDINGS—DATA SOURCES

Public health databases were reviewed for relevant information on elemental mercury-related exposure events. The information presented is from the five relevant sources: 1) ATSDR - Health Consultations and Emergency Response Calls, 2) ATSDR - Hazardous Substances Emergency Events Surveillance, 3) U.S. Coast Guard - National Response Center Database, 4) American Association of Poison Control Centers - National Poison Data System, and 5) Association of Occupational and Environmental Clinics - Pediatric Environmental Health Specialty Units.

Although they did not contain information relevant to this report, the three remaining databases are briefly described: 1) CDC - Clinical Information Service, 2) Environmental Protection Agency - Superfund Sites and the National Priorities List, 3) National Institute for Occupational Safety and Health - -Worker's Home Contamination Study.

5.1. ATSDR - Health Consultations and Emergency Response Calls

ATSDR is the lead federal public health agency for implementing the health provisions of the Comprehensive Environmental Response, Compensation, and Liability Act and its amendments. Under this act, ATSDR evaluates the public health impact of hazardous substances released into the environment. The evaluation of mercury-related events occurs in a number of different ways. ATSDR receives a number of inquiries regarding mercury exposure events. Although some inquiries are not systematically recorded, some are documented as ATSDR Health Consultations (HCs) and others are documented as emergency response calls.

The HCs were reviewed to identify events that document potential mercury exposure to children. Events were selected if there was a completed mercury exposure pathway in air and children were potentially exposed.

During the years 2002 to 2007, ATSDR and its state cooperative agreement partners produced health consultations for 26 events exposed or potentially exposed children to elemental mercury in air (Table 3). These events took place between 2001 and 2006. The degree of hazard posed by these exposures depended on factors such as the concentration of mercury in air and the frequency and duration of exposure. Of these 26 incidents, two children were potentially exposed in more than one location. Fourteen of the 26 (54%) were classified as public health hazards. Although not always mutually exclusive, the location of the exposure event was most frequently described as a home (46%; 12 of 26) or school (42%; 11 of 26). Two of the 26 events (8%) occurred at medical care facilities, one at a daycare center (4%), and one in a car (4%). The source of these mercury exposures included use or storage in schools, release from broken thermometers or sphygmomanometers, off-gassing from flooring containing a mercury catalyst, and an unknown source.

The estimated amount of mercury reported to be released in these 26 exposure events ranged from 9 to 700 ml. The maximum indoor air concentrations of mercury ranged from 0.05 $\mu g/m^3$ to greater than 92 $\mu g/m^3$. Biomonitoring was conducted for children considered exposed in 11 events. The mercury concentrations in blood ranged from below the level of detection (LOD) to 29 $\mu g/L$. The urine concentrations ranged from below the LOD to 18 $\mu g/g$ creatinine. The LOD varied by event. The approximate time interval between exposure and urine collection for testing ranged from 6 to 20 days.

In addition to these HCs, emergency response calls are received from state and local health officials, environmental officials, health care providers, and the general public. From 2000 to 2007, ATSDR's emergency response staff responded to more than 3,000 such inquiries and 459 of them were about mercury events. The majority of the events occurred in residential settings (44%; 203 of 459) or in schools (13%; 60 of 459). These calls were most often made by private citizens (3 1%; 143 of 459); many calls concerned cleaning up mercury-related spills (38%; 175 of 459) or health- related questions about being exposed to mercury (35%; 159 of 459).

Given the relatively few mercury events documented by ATSDR HCs (n=26) compared to the number of mercury-related calls to ATSDR's emergency response staff (n=459), the HCs may not be representative of mercury events nationwide.

5.2. ATSDR - Hazardous Substances Emergency Events Surveillance

ATSDR developed the Hazardous Substances Emergency Events Surveillance (HSEES) system (www.atsdr.cdc.gov/HS/HSEES) to collect data on uncontrolled and/or illegal releases of any hazardous substance [ATSDR 2007a]. Releases of chemicals for more than 72 hours are considered chronic releases and are not captured by HSEES.

A number of U.S. state health departments report chemical releases to HSEES. The data collected include the type of release, the amount of chemical(s) released, the location of the event (private residence, school, etc.), information about any persons with symptoms or injuries ("victims"), and any possible contributing causes that are known. The number of persons exposed during a chemical release is not captured directly in HSEES. However, using victim data and additional information recorded as optional text, one can estimate the number of exposed persons.

The possible contributing causes for the release are categorized as equipment failure, human error, intentional or illegal release, and unknown cause. The human error category includes breaking of or dropping thermometers or other mercury-containing devices or equipment. Intentional or illegal releases include events in which children reportedly played with mercury.

The HSEES events from 2002 through 2006 were included in this compilation if children were potentially exposed to elemental mercury (unpublished HSEES data) (Table 4). Children were defined as persons less than or equal to 19 years of age. Events in which releases were only threatened were omitted. Events were selected if they took place at a private residence, at an elementary or secondary school, or at another location for which children were documented as possibly exposed, injured, or had symptoms associated with mercury exposure.

The HSEES database contained 843 mercury events from 41,709 total events in which hazardous substances were reported to be released from January 2002 through December 2006. Mercury was the only toxicant released in 824 of these events; the remaining 19 mercury events included the release of at least one other hazardous substance. Approximately half of the total mercury events identified (n=409) were classified as potentially exposing children. All 409 events potentially affecting children were mercury only events.

These events were reported from 17 states; only 12 states participated during the entire time period from 2002 through 2006. The remaining states participated for either 2 or 4 years (Table 4).

The 409 events potentially affecting children were most frequently classified as nonvolatilization or spill only events (88%; 360 of 409). Volatilization of mercury was noted in 6 of the 409 events (2%) as air only and in 40 events (10%) as combined spill and air releases. A fire was noted in one of the 409 events (<1%). Although liquid mercury has a relatively low vapor pressure and volatilizes slowly at room temperature, some volatilization was likely in some or all of the events described as spill only. Mercury events occurred most frequently in private households (75%; 307 of 409). The most frequent contributing cause of the event was human error (87%; 357 of 409).

Evacuations were ordered in 68 of the 409 events (17%). The median number evacuated per event was 20 people, with a range from 1 to 1,505 people (data not shown). The total number of people exposed during these 409 events was not captured in HSEES. Five children had elevated levels of mercury in blood/urine. Mercury biomarkers are not routinely reported to HSEES.

Limitations do exist in using HSEES data to report on elemental mercury exposures to children. The HSEES data source is intended to build capacity in state health departments for surveillance of acute releases of hazardous substances and to initiate or improve appropriate prevention activities. HSEES was not designed to enumerate and characterize mercury exposure events affecting children. Information on age is only captured in HSEES if the person reports a symptom or requires medical follow- up; for this reason, H SEES data are likely to underestimate the number of children exposed. The magnitude of exposure is difficult to determine given that the amount of mercury released or spilled is often reported as a range rather than a specific quantity. Therefore, a reliable calculation of the average amount of mercury released is not possible. Lastly, the reporting of mercury-related events to HSEES is uneven across the participating states. States with mercury exposure prevention initiatives may report more mercury-related events than states without mercury initiatives (see Supplemental Material) [MDEQ 2007; MPCA 2006]. For example, the emphasis that Michigan and Minnesota placed on preventing mercury exposure may have increased the awareness and reporting of such events. Lastly, HSEES reports acute releases; incidents in which mercury exposure continued for an extended period of time are not included.

5.3. U.S. Coast Guard - National Response Center Database

Under federal law, the release or spill of one pound (33 ml, approximately 2 tablespoons) or more of mercury into the environment must be reported to the federal government (40 Code of Federal Regulations [CFR] 302.4). The primary contact for reporting these events is the National Response Center (NRC), operated by the U.S. Coast Guard for the National Response Team established under the National Contingency Plan for Oil and Hazardous Substances Releases (40 CFR 300) (www.nrc.uscg.mil/nrcback.html).

NRC receives between 25,000 and 30,000 reports of pollution incidents and response drills each year. To identify events for this report, data for the years 2002 through 2007 were downloaded from the NRC Web site and queried using statistical software SAS 9.1. Mercury-related events were identified by a) a Chemical Abstracts Service registry number recorded as "00743 9-97-6" (denoting mercury was released) or b) the word "mercury" reported in the name of the material released, in the description of the incident, in the description of remedial actions, or in the additional information provided. A total of 825 events met this definition between 2002 and 2007 (Table 5). Actual exposures may have taken place prior to the year in which the spill was reported.

To assess the number of events in which children were potentially exposed, two additional searches were conducted on the 825 mercury events. First, school and daycare settings were always selected as locations where children were potentially exposed by searching for the terms "school" or "daycare" in the incident description, in the location of the incident, or in the additional information field. Second, the description of the incident and the additional information fields were queried for a series of 11 words or parts of words that represent terms commonly used to describe children (i.e., infant, toddler, child, adolescent). Of the mercury incidents reported over the 6-year period, 113 (14%; 113 of 825) were events in which children were potentially exposed.

Table 5 summarizes the number of mercury events and the number of such events in which children were likely exposed. The location of the incident was not reported in 45 (40%) of the 113 events in which children were likely exposed. A few events noted more than one exposure location. When only a street address was given, the category "other" was used to describe the event location (Table 6).

To compare the amounts of mercury released in different events, the quantity was expressed as ml of mercury. The amount of mercury released varied from less than 1 ml to approximately 1,900 ml. For example, a fire occurred in one event, and the event released approximately 200 ml of mercury at a school. No information was provided on whether children were present during the release.

Among the 113 events that potentially exposed children, five people were injured and five people were hospitalized. Whether the five persons injured were the same five persons who were hospitalized is unclear. The states reporting the most incidents that potentially exposed children were Kentucky, Michigan, Mississippi, and Ohio (Figure 2). In 27 events persons were evacuated. These evacuations took place in a number of locations, including homes and schools.

NRC reports contain the initial conditions of each event and are self reported, often by the spiller. Details often are not known or not volunteered in these initial reports, which results in reporting errors and missing information. Furthermore, mercury spills that draw media attention and state-based mercury initiatives may result in increased and more thorough reporting. The type of mercury is not always specified, leading to potential misclassification of mercury exposures. Since the NRC does not systematically collect the age of persons exposed, the information on children was only present when volunteered. Any analysis of these events is limited by these factors.

5.4. American Association of Poison Control Centers - National Poison Data System

The American Association of Poison Control Centers (AAPCC) National Poison Data System represents information uploaded in near real-time from 61 of 62 U.S. Poison Control Centers__(*www.aapcc.org/dnn/NPDS /tabid/65/Default.aspx*). Reporting is passive and voluntary, occurring when a caller reports a known or suspected chemical exposure. Poison Control Center specialists collect basic demographic data, information about the chemical agent and exposure route, and any reported clinical effects associated with the case. Depending on the nature of the call, a specialist chooses from a pre-established list of chemical agents and selects signs and symptoms from a list of 131 clinical effects. AAPCC classifies persons 19 years of age and younger as children.

Between 2002 and 2006 the AAPCC received approximately 12 million calls. Of these total calls 15,739 were mercury-related calls (Table 7) that were not associated with broken thermometers. The majority of these calls concerned elemental mercury exposure events (9 1%; 14,378 of 15,739). The calls concerning children (n=6,396) made up 44% (6,396 of 14,378) of the elemental mercury calls. Although many calls specified dermal exposure or ingestion, such exposures also included the potential for inhalational exposure. Michigan and Illinois recorded the most calls to AAPCC for potential childhood mercury exposures (Figure 2).

AAPCC also receives a large number of calls regarding broken mercury thermometers. The types of mercury thermometers recorded include: general formulation, basal, high/low, oral fever, baby rectal, yellow back glass, and mercury metal. Since 2002, the calls for mercury thermometer exposures have continued to decrease (Table 8). In 2002, there were 10,108 calls regarding children exposed to mercury thermometers. The number of calls decreased to 2,896 in 2006.

Each year between 2002 and 2005, 93% or more of the non-thermometer-related mercury exposures in children were coded as unintentional. In 2006, the percentage of unintentional exposures dropped to 80% (758 of 948). This decrease probably resulted from a single incident in which AAPCC received 157 calls regarding adolescent children intentionally exposed to elemental mercury. All 157 calls were made on the same day from the same state.

AAPCC also records the anticipated health effects of the exposure. Effects are categorized as minor, moderate, major, not-followed, and unable to follow [Bronstein et al. 2007]. AAPCC describes minor effects as those with minimally bothersome symptoms and generally resolve rapidly. Moderate effects are more pronounced or more systemic in nature. Major effects as those that may be life-threatening or result in disability or disfigurement. Calls are not followed when the exposure was minimal to nontoxic in nature, the amount of the contaminant released was insignificant, or the route of exposure was unlikely to result in a clinical effect. Between 2002 and 2006, most non-thermometer (93%; 5,966 of 6,396) and thermometer (98%; 30,287 of 30,891)-related calls were reported as not-followed. Five of the 6,396 calls (<1%) regarding children were about events that may have had a major effect. All five calls were non-thermometer-related. No major effects were reported among mercury thermometer-related calls.

A strength of the AAPCC data is that calls are classified as those representing an actual human exposure event or classified as other calls, such as those seeking only information. The limitations of the data relate to the passive and incomplete nature of the reporting and the general lack of environmental or human exposure monitoring. In addition, how many of the calls report separate exposure events is unclear; for example, a school-based exposure may prompt a number of concerned parents to call the AAPCC. Media attention regarding a mercury exposure event and state-based mercury initiatives (see Supplemental Material) probably influence public awareness and the reporting of mercury events to the AAPCC.

5.5. Association of Occupational and Environmental Clinics - Pediatric Environmental Health Specialty Units

The Association of Occupational and Environmental Clinics maintains the network of Pediatric Environmental Health Specialty Units (PEHSU) to provide consultation to health care professionals and parents for environmental health concerns affecting children and their families_(www.aoec.org/PEHSU.htm). Eleven of the 13 PEHSU clinics are located in the United States.

Prior to 2004, the PEHSU consultation data were not easily queried. Therefore, only events recorded for the period from April 2004 through September 2007 were queried. The database does not differentiate among calls about elemental, inorganic, and organic mercury. The database includes age, gender, date of call, and PEHSU region. Of the 2,910 calls to PEHSU between 2004 and 2007, 242 were mercury exposure calls. One hundred twenty (50%) concerned potentially exposed boys, 93 (38%) concerned girls, and the sex of the remaining 29 (12%) was not identified. The age of the child was recorded for 225 calls; the majority of these calls concerned children less than 7 years old (Figure 3). The larger percentage of calls concerning younger children may result from the PEHSU focus on young children.

Since April 2006, the database also has included the role of the caller (parent, physician, etc.) and the exposure location, identified as daycare, home, public area, school, waste site, or unknown. PEHSU received 145 calls during the 18-month period from April 2006 through September 2007. In 108 of the 145 calls (74%), the parent of the potentially exposed child made the call. The most common exposure locations identified were homes and daycare facilities (Figure 4).

These data are limited by passive and incomplete reporting and the general lack of environmental or human exposure monitoring data. In addition, how many of these calls may pertain to the same event is unclear. Media attention regarding a mercury exposure event and the implementation of state-based mercury initiatives (see Supplemental Material) are likely to influence public awareness and the reporting of mercury events to PEHSU.

5.6. CDC - Clinical Information Service

CDC's National Center for Health Marketing collects information from calls made to the agency's consolidated call center (1-800-CDC-INFO), a service that delivers health information to consumers, health care providers, and other professionals (www.emergency.cdc.gov/coca/800cdcinfo.asp). The information collected is limited to the question asked and the standardized (prepared) answer provided. Detailed information about the specifics of the call is not collected. Also, more than one prepared answer is given to a caller when more than one issue is raised, and each of these question/answer combinations is counted individually.

No information is recorded on the number of persons potentially affected by the event that led to the call. Overall, the CDC-INFO data were not sufficient to characterize the source, location, and distribution of mercury exposures. Therefore, these data were not considered further in this report.

5.7. Environmental Protection Agency - Superfund Sites and the National Priorities List

U.S. Environmental Protection Agency (EPA) is a federal agency that conducts environmental science, research, education, and site assessment efforts. The mission of the EPA is to protect human health and welfare and the environment. Two databases related to the EPA Superfund program were considered for obtaining mercury event information for this report: the Superfund Information System site (http://cfpub.epa.gov/supercpad/cursites/srchsites.cfm); and the National Priority List (NPL) search site (http://www.epa.gov/superfund/sites/query/advquery.htm). Both databases contain information about specific sites assessed by the Superfund program.

The data on sites containing mercury in various media are available by site name, location, and NPL status. The information available includes an assessment regarding whether human exposure occurred and whether the exposure was contained. The above databases provide no quantifiable information on the amount of mercury released or the number of children potentially exposed. In a proportion of these sites, linking site related data from EPA and other agencies (e.g., ATSDR) might provide additional information. This linking was not feasible for this report, given the required cost in time and resources. Therefore, neither EPA database was considered further in this report.

5.8. National Institute for Occupational Safety and Health - Worker's Home Contamination Study

The mission of the National Institute for Occupational Safety and Health (NIOSH) is to protect worker health and safety. Thus, the majority of NIOSH work concerns adult exposures in the workplace. However, exposure data related to children are occasionally included if the workplace is frequented by children (e.g., schools and some health care clinics).

In addition, the actions of adult workers may affect the exposure and health of children they encounter outside the workplace. In 1995, NIOSH published a report to Congress on the contamination of workers' homes [NIOSH 1995]. This report also summarized the information available on the exposure of workers' children to mercury. In this report, the airborne concentration of mercury in the homes of workers ranged from 0.02 $\mu g/m^3$ to 50 $\mu g/m^3$. Although potentially relevant, the information in this report predates the time period reviewed by the workgroup (2002– 2007) and does not meet the selection criteria for this report. Therefore, it was not considered further in this report.

6. FINDINGS—LITERATURE REVIEW

During the years 2002 to 2007, 10 published reports met the criteria for inclusion described in the methods section (7.3. Literature Review) (Table 9) [AzzizBaumgartner et al. 2007; Baughman 2006; CDC 2005a, b; Cherry et al. 2002; CNN 2003; Gattineni et al. 2007; Gordon 2004; Hryhorczuk et al. 2006; Johnson 2004; Tominack et al. 2002]

These 10 publications reported 13 events that exposed approximately 1,393 children between 1998 and 2004 (Table 9). The year of the exposure was not reported for two of these events. The children exposed ranged in age from 2 to 18 years old. Exposures took place in homes, cars, schools, and school buses. In eight events a child obtained mercury by stealing. Mercury was stolen from a school in 6 of the 13 events (46%), once from a dental office (8%), and once from an industrial site (8%). The mercury was subsequently dispersed or sold to other children. When reported, the estimated amount of mercury spilled/released ranged from 9 to 701 ml. The events reporting the largest releases typically occurred after children stole mercury from an industrial site (approximately 701 ml of mercury released) or a school (30–40 ml of mercury released). When mercury was taken from a school, children typically played with the material at school and then at home, producing exposures in multiple locations.

In four additional reports, the exposure resulted from mercury found in the home. The sources of mercury included mercury-containing devices, prior spills, and mercury stored in the home. The largest potential source for home-based exposure was mercury spills from gas regulators. One publication estimated that mercury was spilled in 1,363 homes [Hryhorczuk et al. 2006]. Although many children were likely exposed, information is not available to determine how many children were actually exposed in these 1,363 homes.

Although the ages of the children exposed ranged from 2 to 18 years old, adolescent youth obtained mercury more frequently than other age groups. Depending upon clinical symptoms and the availability of laboratory tests, many of these children were tested for biomarkers of inorganic mercury exposure. The results ranged from less than 0.20 to greater than 1,000 µg/L in urine and from less than 4 to 295 µg/L in blood. Neither urine nor blood mercury levels correlate well with the presence or severity of symptoms [Cherry et al. 2002; Gattineni et al. 2007; Tominack et al. 2002].

7. FINDINGS—EXPOSURE SCENARIOS

To further describe the types of elemental mercury exposures that occur, three categories of exposure scenarios are presented. The intent of these scenarios is to illustrate the nature and public health impact of these events. Each scenario describes the source of exposure and provides additional information about the number of children affected. Some of these scenarios also illustrate how nonspecific symptoms combined with an environmental exposure history can help medical providers identify mercury exposures.

The first two categories are scenarios in the home and those at school, two common locations for childhood elemental mercury exposures. The third category includes exposures at other locations, such as medical clinics and property that was not adequately remediated. In some scenarios, elemental mercury is carried or tracked to multiple locations, making the primary exposure location difficult to specify.

These cases are examples of exposure scenarios that have occurred. The characteristics of individual exposure scenarios and associated health outcomes are not generalizable.

7.1. Exposure at Home

The sources of exposure in the home include mercury-containing devices, cultural or ceremonial uses of mercury, intentionally heating elemental mercury, and unknowingly tracking mercury home from the workplace. These examples are illustrated in the scenarios below.

Mercury-Containing Devices. Mercury exposure most commonly results from spills associated with broken thermometers, barometers, and other medical or scientific instruments used in the home. The most common exposure scenario involves mercury from broken thermometers. In the vast majority of such cases, the reported mercury vapor levels are low. Baughman [2006] reported that broken mercury thermometers rarely result in mercury vapor levels above 1 $\mu g/m^3$. It is important to clean up all such releases properly [Chrysochoou et al. 2003].

In a Swiss example, an 11-month-old infant had a medical evaluation for nonspecific symptoms, including restlessness, swollen hands and feet (with skin desquamation), profuse sweating, and repeated biting of objects or his own hands [Chrysochoou et al. 2003]. During the following 3 months, the infant failed to thrive and developed tachycardia and arterial hypertension. After hospitalization and an extensive medical evaluation, the parents were asked about mercury exposure. The parents confirmed that 4 weeks prior to the initial onset of symptoms a broken thermometer had spilled mercury onto a carpet and was subsequently vacuumed. Based on the symptoms, physical findings, and environmental exposure history, acrodynia was diagnosed. Over time the child's symptoms resolved and his growth and development returned to normal.

In a similar incident, a 9-year-old boy presented to a hospital with lethargy, limb pain, and unsteadiness [Rennie et al. 1999]. The child's physical examination showed mild facial weakness, areflexia, ataxia, and impaired sensation. He also developed hypertension. An investigation revealed that 3 months earlier the boy dismantled a mercury-containing sphygmomanometer in his bedroom and spilled mercury onto his bed and carpet. Although the amounts vary, sphygmomanometers typically contain 11 ml of mercury [Caravati et al. 2008]. Upon discovery of the mercury spill, his parents unsuccessfully attempted to clean it up by vacuuming. Subsequently, officials from the health department had to remove the bedding, carpets, and clothing from the room. A mercury vapor absorbing filter system was used in the bedroom for 3 months to remove residual mercury vapors. Over the next 6 months, the child slowly returned to this premorbid state.

Reports have been made of other elemental mercury exposure sources in the home, although these are less frequently encountered. Prior to 1961, most residential natural gas meters and pressure regulators were placed inside homes in some parts of the United States. Each gas regulator contained about 10 ml of mercury. After 1961, alternative technology became available and the industry began placing regulators outdoors. As a result, gas utility companies began relocating meters and pressure regulators to locations outside the residence during the 1980s. In 2000, a homeowner near Chicago discovered mercury in the house's basement after the gas meter and regulator were relocated. This homeowner called the regional poison control center, initiating a response that eventually involved 2 states, 4 natural gas companies, 6 state agencies, 2 federal agencies, and 500,000 homes and businesses [ATSDR 2001a; Hryhorczuk et al. 2006]. The mercury was most likely spilled in the homes during relocation of the regulator to an outdoor location.

To assess the potential for other mercury spills related to the relocation of these gas regulators, a taskforce was formed with representatives from federal, state, and local public health agencies, as well as local government, medical care facilities, and three utility companies. The taskforce developed protocols to evaluate homes and characterize the threat. If data indicated that concentrations in the homes exceeded 1 µg/m^3, cleanup was initiated and residents were offered free clinical evaluations. If the concentration exceeded 10 µg/m^3, the occupants were offered relocation (pending cleanup) and urged to seek clinical evaluations [ATSDR 2001a].

According to one analysis completed after the response was over, the likelihood of residential mercury contamination exceeding the cleanup level after gas regulator removal ranged from 0.9/1,000 homes to 4.3/1,000 homes and varied by the gas company [Hryhorczuk et al. 2006]. This response has provided a template for similar problems in other metropolitan areas in recent years. This response also provided the basis for a field operations guide later developed by EPA.

Cultural or Ceremonial Uses. Some practitioners of certain Caribbean and Latin American religions, such as Voodoo, Santeria, Palo, and Espiritismo, use mercury ceremonially [EPA 2002; Johnson 1999; Newby et al. 2006; Wendroff 2005; Zayas and Ozuah 1996]. Ceremonial uses of mercury include applying it to the skin, adding it to candles, or sprinkling it around the home. These practices can potentially expose practitioners and their families. Because mercury contamination in the home can persist for years, ceremonial use of mercury in the home could expose future occupants and their children, contributing to health disparities in these populations.

Previous reports document the ceremonial use of mercury in neighborhoods whose residents are largely Hispanic [JSI 2003; Ozuah et al. 2003; Rogers et al. 2008; Rogers et al. 2007; Zayas and Ozuah 1996]. The John Snow, Inc. Center for Environmental Health Studies [2003] reported a survey of 898 persons, most of whom had Latino or Caribbean backgrounds. In this survey, 344 of the 898 people (38%) reported that they used or knew someone who used mercury for religious, spiritual, or health purposes. Garetano et al. [2008] found that mercury vapor levels were higher among residential common areas belonging to communities likely to use mercury for cultural practices than control areas where cultural mercury use is uncommon. However, all mercury vapor levels observed by Garetano et al. [2008] were below the ATSDR minimum risk level for chronic inhalation of metallic mercury [ATSDR 1999]. An exposure assessment by Rogers et al. [2007] tested the urine mercury levels of 306 children who lived in an area where elemental mercury was commonly sold for ritualistic use. Although no relationship between ritualistic use and mercury exposure was evident, Rogers et al. [2007] concluded that potential health hazards remain when mercury is readily available. In a similar study, urine mercury levels were measured in 100 children that resided in an area where elemental mercury was commonly sold for religious practices. Five percent of these children had urine mercury levels above 5 µg/L [Ozuah et al. 2003; Zayas and Ozuah 1996].

Heating Elemental Mercury. On rare occasions, there have been reports of heating elemental mercury in the home. As noted previously, heating mercury results in much higher (potentially lethal) concentrations in air, especially in enclosed spaces such as a home [Putman and Madden 1972; Solis et al. 2000; Taueg et al. 1992].

In one published report, six children were exposed to mercury vapor when the parents attempted to extract gold ore while heating elemental mercury in a poorly ventilated kitchen [Solis et al. 2000]. All six children had elevated urinary mercury levels (range 45 – 575 µg/L). The two children in the kitchen were exposed to the highest mercury vapor levels. These two children developed respiratory symptoms within a few hours and were thought to have pneumonia until the environmental exposure history was obtained. One child died of respiratory failure and the other child recovered.

From the Workplace to the Home. The NIOSH [1995] Worker's Home Contamination Study found that airborne mercury concentrations in the homes of workers ranged from 0.02 µg/m^3 to 50 µg/m^3. The ATSDR recommended limit in the breathing zone of a home after an elemental mercury spill is <1 µg/m^3 [ATSDR 2001a]. Although the NIOSH study predates the time period analyzed for the current report, the findings suggest that workers can inadvertently track mercury from the workplace into the home.

7.2. Exposure at School

The most common elemental mercury sources in schools are mercury stored in science laboratories, mercury found in broken instruments, and mercury brought to school from other locations. In addition, some gymnasium floors contain a mercury catalyst that can release mercury vapor into the air. Case reports to illustrate these two scenarios are presented below.

Student Misuse of Mercury. During the winter of 2004, 854 students at a middle school in Nevada were exposed to elemental mercury [Azziz-Baumgartner et al. 2007; Burgess 2007]. A student found a container of mercury in a storage shed and took it home for several weeks. The student subsequently brought approximately 60 ml of the mercury to school, where several students played with it (e.g., threw it at each other, rolled it on the floor).

Only one third of the 60 ml of mercury was recovered. Mercury vapor levels in the school were highest near the locker rooms (50 $\mu g/m^3$). Indoor mercury vapor levels were higher than background levels measured in other Nevada buildings (0.0 10– 0.040 $\mu g/m^3$) Of the 854 students potentially exposed, 200 completed an exposure history and provided urine samples. In general, the creatinine-adjusted urine mercury levels were below the Azziz-Baumgartner et al. [2007] reported comparison value (3.99 $\mu g/L$). The mean urine mercury level for all tested students was 0.36 $\mu g/L$ (range 0.14–11.4 $\mu g/L$).

Students who reported exposure to the mercury (n=66) had significantly higher urine mercury levels than those who did not. Those who touched the mercury and/or got it on their clothes (n=64) also had significantly higher urine mercury levels than those who did not. Self-reported symptoms were rare and no students required emergency medical treatment.

Mercury Vapors from School Flooring. In most situations, children are exposed to elemental mercury as a result of misuse or mishandling of mercury or mercury- containing devices. However, from the 1960s to the 1980s, many schools throughout the United States installed synthetic floors that contained a mercury catalyst. One manufacturer claimed to have installed more than 25 million pounds of polyurethane flooring over the past 40 years. A mercury-containing catalyst was used in the polyurethane formulation that formed the floor covering; the finished product typically contained 0.1% to 0.2% mercury [ATSDR 2003]. These surfaces slowly release elemental mercury vapor, particularly from damaged areas. State health departments in Ohio [ATSDR 2003], Michigan, and Oregon [ATSDR 2003, 2004, 2006] performed initial public health investigations. The airborne concentrations of mercury in gymnasium settings vary. One school district reported mercury vapor from 0.79 to 1.6 $\mu g/m^3$ [ATSDR 2003]. Another school reported 0.042 to 0.050 $\mu g/m^3$ in the breathing zone [ATSDR 2004]. The variation is likely a factor of many attributes, including the environmental sampling equipment used, the size of the floor, relative damage to the flooring material, and ventilation.

7.3. Exposures in Other Locations

Mercury exposures can also occur in medical facilities and buildings where mercury was previously used. Sources include prior mercury spills, mercury stored on abandoned property, and mercury found in medical or dental offices. In some cases, mercury is carried or tracked into multiple locations, making a primary exposure location difficult to identify.

Prior Industrial Mercury Contamination. In most situations the reuse of industrial property does not result in childhood mercury exposure. However, an increase in the redevelopment of industrial property for other uses increases the chance of this scenario occurring in the future.

One such exposure scenario occurred in Hoboken, New Jersey [Orloff et al. 1997]. A building that was formerly used to manufacture mercury vapor lamps was converted to private condominiums. After moving into the building, residents reported seeing drops of mercury on their oven and kitchen countertops. Investigations revealed pools of mercury in the subflooring and corresponding elevated indoor air mercury levels throughout the building.

Investigators measured the urinary mercury concentrations of 29 residents of the building, 6 of whom were children under the age of 9 years old. The urine levels ranged from 4.8 to 133 µg/g creatinine. All occupants of the building and their uncontaminated possessions were relocated. Because of the extensive mercury contamination, the decontamination efforts were unsuccessful and the building was eventually demolished.

A similar situation occurred in a Franklinville, New Jersey, daycare facility opened in 2004. The daycare facility was located in a building that previously manufactured mercury-containing thermometers. The daycare center was closed in 2006 after environmental samples from areas occupied by children revealed elevated levels of elemental mercury in wipe samples (<0.02 to 0.25 µg/wipe) and in air samples (7.0 to 11.4 µg/m^3) [ATSDR 2007b].

After the daycare closed, federal and state agencies tested urine samples from 91 children and 13 staff members for mercury. A value of 5 µg/g creatinine was used for comparison purposes. Approximately one third of the children had a urine mercury level greater than the comparison value at the initial round of screening. Serial testing confirmed that the elevated urine mercury levels decreased over time to levels below the comparison value. This evidence indicated that the mercury exposure pathway was interrupted following the daycare's closure. The medical records of 22 of the participants who provided urine samples were reviewed. There was no evidence of mercury related health effects in the medical records of 21 of the 22 participants. For one child, the medical records showed some evidence of conditions potentially related, but not specific for, mercury exposure. This child's health conditions resolved several months after enrollment ended [ATSDR 2007b].

In addition to being exposed by the reuse of inadequately remediated industrial property, children have been exposed to elemental mercury stored on abandoned industrial property. The following is an example in which children scavenged elemental mercury from an old industrial site. This scenario also shows that the three location-based exposure categories are not mutually exclusive.

Two teenagers in Texarkana, Arkansas, removed a large amount of mercury from an abandoned neon sign plant [Lowry et al. 1999]. The mercury was estimated to weigh between 23 and 100 pounds (770 to 3,300 ml). One of the teenagers took mercury home and gave some of it to other children. Health officials investigating this incident found mercury contamination in 12 residences, a convenience store, and a school classroom. Residents of several highly contaminated homes were relocated during remediation. One house and an apartment were so contaminated that remediation was not possible. Both structures were demolished. For persons who had both a urinary and blood mercury test, initial urinary concentrations ranged as high 66.6 µg/g creatinine, and blood mercury concentrations ranged as high as 104 µg/L. Neurobehavioral assessment of the eight exposed individuals failed to establish a relationship between mercury exposures and test results.

Mercury-Containing Medical Equipment. Mishandling of mercury and mercury- containing medical equipment can occur in medical and dental offices. In one such example, mercury was spilled from a sphygmomanometer [ATSDR 2001b]. A patient who observed the attempted cleanup reported the incident to the Poison Control Center. The state health department and EPA responded, measuring breathing zone concentrations of mercury between 45 and 50 $\mu g/m^3$ in some areas. Visible beads and small pools of mercury were also observed in the clinic, which served both adults and children. Patients and staff were evacuated from the contaminated areas, and a professional environmental contractor was hired to carry out remedial activities.

8. LIMITATIONS

The information available on childhood mercury exposures varies among the data sources reviewed for this report. As noted previously, each data source contains its own limitations. These data sources were designed to document hazardous releases of toxic chemicals; information on children who were potentially exposed is not routinely collected. Furthermore, the duplication and inconsistent reporting of events between data sources and even within data sources (e.g., among states reporting to HSEES) make any estimate of the national incidence of mercury exposure to children unreliable.

Concerns regarding personal responsibility for causing a spill or having to clean up a spill may influence the quality and completeness of the information reported. Spills in private residences may be under reported because the residents are unaware of the health hazard and the need to report spills more than 1 pound (33 ml, approximately 2 tablespoons) to the NRC. Published case reports and case series often provide exposure and health outcome information but are limited by reporting bias, retrospective data collection, and imprecise estimates of exposure dose and duration. For these reasons, the frequencies described are not generalizable. In addition, the published literature is likely biased toward reporting worst-case scenarios, as opposed to the more typical exposures that do not cause symptoms or attract attention.

Case reports from the literature provide more information about risk factors, exposure scenarios, and associated health outcomes. The specifics relate to the individual cases and are not representative of all exposure scenarios.

Despite their limitations, the data sources reviewed in this report are the best available data sources on acute exposures to hazardous substances in the United States. Excluding events that were reported prior to 2002, this report provides an overview of the current information available on elemental mercury exposure events and provides examples of potential exposure scenarios.

9. DISCUSSION

The ATSDR\CDC Mercury Workgroup was formed to address the Congressional directive that ATSDR assess the extent of children's exposure to mercury from former industrial sites and other sources nationwide. The specific objectives included: 1) identify the sources associated with elemental mercury exposure in children and 2) describe the location, demographics, and proportion of children exposed or potentially exposed to elemental mercury in the United States. These objectives are further described in sections 12.1 and 12.2.

9.1. Identifying Exposure Sources Associated with Elemental Mercury

This review of data sources and scientific literature found that children are most frequently exposed to mercury when mercury is mishandled or when people improperly clean up spilled mercury.

Children are potentially exposed to mercury that is scavenged, collected, and pooled from sources such as school science laboratories, electrical or medical equipment, and industrial sites [Azziz-Baumgartner et al. 2007; Baughman 2006; CDC 2005a, b; Gordon 2004; Tominack et al. 2002].

Exposure to small spills from broken thermometers represents the most frequent scenario, based upon reports retrieved from AAPCC. Caravati et al. [2008] reported that mercury thermometer exposures reported to AAPCC declined 48% from 2001 through 2005. The increased use of mercury free thermometers may have led to this decline. In 2000, 11 national retailers jointly issued a press release in which they pledged to stop selling mercury thermometers. In addition, the nation's largest manufacturer of mercury thermometers announced plans to stop producing them [Goldstein 2000]. In 2008, the Interstate Mercury Education and Reduction Clearinghouse, a program of the Northeast Waste Management Officials' Association, reported an 11% reduction in the sale of mercury-containing products from 2001 to 2004 [IMERC 2008].

Although the sales of some mercury-containing products have decreased, sales of the compact fluorescent lightbulb (CFL) are increasing. The CFL is an EPA Energy Star recommended product that is an effective way to reduce energy use. However, each CFL contains a small amount of mercury, which makes disposal in regular refuse problematic. Given the potential cumulative hazard from breaking a large number of CFLs, or the disposal of large numbers of CFLs in landfills, the public must learn about the need for proper disposal and have easy access to appropriate disposal facilities.

9.2. Describing the Location, Demographics, and Proportion of Children Affected

Mercury exposures are divided into three primary categories based on location. Ordered by relative frequency, these exposure categories include exposures that occur 1) in the home, 2) at school, and 3) at other locations such as inadequately remediated industrial properties or medical facilities. In all of these locations, the primary exposure pathway of concern is through inhalation of elemental mercury. Children may play with and disperse mercury in more than one location such as a home or school. Once dispersed, the droplets may volatilize and contaminate indoor air. Inhaling mercury vapor may go unrecognized, as it is colorless and odorless.

The demographics and proportion of U.S. children affected by these exposures is not directly quantifiable using the various data sources reviewed. Most data sources that collect information on the release of hazardous substances do not systematically collect information on the persons affected. The typical exposure scenario involves relatively small amounts of mercury without reports of human illness. Neither urine nor blood mercury levels correlate well with the presence or severity of symptoms [Cherry et al. 2002; Gattineni et al. 2007; Tominack et al. 2002]. Elevated mercury vapor levels are documented at times, but health effects are rarely reported after small mercury spills (e.g., broken fever thermometer). Regardless, one must clean up even small spills properly and avoid improper actions such as tracking and vacuuming. Caravati et al. [2008] did not identify any clinical toxicity after small spills that were properly cleaned up.

Although the extent of mercury use in the home for religious purposes is not well characterized, such use may lead to chronic mercury exposure among those who use it in this manner and for subsequent occupants of the contaminated homes. Some evidence suggests that attempting to ban mercury could drive its use and sales underground, making the risks of using mercury and the benefits of mercury-free alternatives difficult for local health officials to communicate [Riley et al. 2001]. The individuals affected are most likely to be members of minority populations, raising concerns about environmental injustice in these communities.

10. CONCLUSIONS

Although other efforts have focused on chronic mercury exposures that are beyond the control of most individuals, this report focuses on exposures to elemental mercury that are clearly preventable. Reducing the population's exposure to heavy metals such as mercury, as measured by blood and urine concentrations, supports the Healthy People 2010 recommendations [DHHS 2000].

Although credibly estimating the frequency of elemental mercury exposures among children in the United States is not possible, such exposures are occurring. These incidents typically result from the misuse of mercury-containing equipment or a lack of knowledge regarding the hazard. Exposure events most frequently occur in the home and school and are typically a result of the misuse of mercury or mercury- containing equipment. The typical exposure scenario involves relatively small amounts of mercury (e.g., broken mercury thermometer) without reports of human illness. Elevated mercury vapor levels have been documented after small spills, but demonstrable health effects are rarely identified or reported. However, in some situations medical providers have identified mercury exposures by taking an environmental exposure history while evaluating children for nonspecific symptoms [Chrysochoou et al. 2003; Solis et al. 2000].

As the amount of mercury released increases, so does the risk for harmful exposure. Better coordination of exposure and health information is needed to determine the number of children potentially harmed by larger mercury spills. Regardless, all spills should be cleaned up properly. The EPA website titled, "Spills, Disposal and Site Cleanup" provides useful information on how to appropriately clean up mercury spills (http://www.epa.gov/hg/spills/).

Initiatives that affect the number of children exposed have focused on reducing or removing mercury from consumer products, eliminating mercury from school science laboratories, and educating the public and school officials about its toxicity. These targeted initiatives have great potential. For example, Indiana, Minnesota, Michigan, and Wisconsin have mercury-awareness programs that provide advice and resources to the public regarding mercury toxicity, cleanup after spills, and proper disposal of mercury. Supplemental information on initiatives that may reduce exposure frequency is presented in the Appendix. This section provides information on some current mercury prevention initiatives. This section also describes a number of useful resources for obtaining additional information on mercury hazards and preventing mercury exposures.

In several states (e.g., Michigan), schools are required to eliminate mercury use in the classroom and in the school nurse's office [Legislative Council 2001]. As with removing mercury from thermometers, primary prevention efforts that focus on decreasing the availability of other mercury sources offer the best hope for protecting children (see Supplemental Material). In addition, eliminating mercury sources also eliminates potentially expensive cleanup costs. Although mercury thermometers and other mercury-containing equipment are being phased out, many containers and products containing mercury remain in schools, medical facilities, and homes, which could result in future childhood exposures.

11. REFERENCES

Aposhian, H. V., Bruce, D. C., Alter, W., Dart, R. C., Hurlbut, K. M., Aposhian, M. M. (1992). Urinary mercury after administration of 2,3 - dimercaptopropane- 1 -sulfonic acid: Correlation with dental amalgam score. *FASEBJ, 6(7)*, 2472–2476.

[ATSDR] Agency for Toxic Substances and Disease Registry. (1998). Public health assessment: Grand Street Mercury Site, Hoboken, Hudson County, New Jersey. Available from: http://www.atsdr.cdc.gov/ HAC/pha/grand/gsm_toc.html [accessed 3 December 2007].

[ATSDR] Agency for Toxic Substances and Disease Registry. (1999). Toxicological profile for mercury. Available from: http://www.atsdr. cdc.gov/toxprofiles/tp46.pdf [accessed 3 December 2007].

[ATSDR] Agency for Toxic Substances and Disease Registry. (2001a). Health consultation: Residential mercury spills from gas regulators in Illinois (a/k/a NICOR) MT. Prospect, Lake County, Illinois. Available from: http://www.atsdr.cdc.gov/HAC/pha/resmerc/nic_p1.html [accessed 1 December 2008].

[ATSDR] Agency for Toxic Substances and Disease Registry. (2001b). Health consultation: West Grand Boulevard mercury spill. Available from: *http://www.michigan.gov/documents/West_Grand_Blvd_(Blood_ Pressure_Instrument)_1* 02584_7.pdf [accessed 1 May 2008].

[ATSDR] Agency for Toxic Substances and Disease Registry. (2001c). Summary report hair analysis panel discussion: Exploring the state of the science. Available from: *http://www.atsdr.cdc.gov/hac/hair_analysis/ index.html* [accessed 5 September 2008].

[ATSDR] Agency for Toxic Substances and Disease Registry. (2003). Health consultation: Mercury exposures from 3M Tartan brand floors—Westerville Schools, Westerville, Franklin County, Ohio. Available from: http://www.atsdr.cdc.gov/HAC/PHA/westerville/wes_toc.html [accessed 3 December 2007].

[ATSDR] Agency for Toxic Substances and Disease Registry. (2004). Health consultation: Mid-Michigan mercury floor, Middleton Gratiot County, Michigan. Available from: *http://www.michigan.gov /documents/ Middleton_(mercury_in_flooring)_102577_7.pdf* [accessed 3 December 2007].

[ATSDR] Agency for Toxic Substances and Disease Registry. (2006). Health consultation: Salem-Keizer school district 3M flooring - Salem, OR. Available from: *http://www.atsdr.cdc.gov/HAC/PHA/SalemKeizer SchoolDistrict/SalemKeizerSchoolHC071206.pdf* [accessed 15 February 2008].

[ATSDR] Agency for Toxic Substances and Disease Registry. (2007a). Hazardous Substances Emergency Events Surveillance. Available from: http://www.atsdr.cdc.gov/HS/HSEES [accessed 12 October 2007].

[ATSDR] Agency for Toxic Substances and Disease Registry. (2007b). Health consultation: Mercury exposure investigation using serial urine testing and medical records review, Kiddie Kollege. Available from: http://www.state.nj.us/health/eoh/cehsweb/kiddiekollege/documents/kiddi ekollegehc.pdf [accessed 3 December 2007].

Azziz-Baumgartner, E., Luber, G., Schurz-Rogers, H., Backer, L., Belson, M. & Kieszak, S., et al. (2007). Exposure assessment of a mercury spill in a Nevada school--2004. *Clin Toxicol (Phila), 45*(4), 391–395.

Barregard, L., Sallsten, G. & Conradi, N. (1999). Tissue levels of mercury determined in a deceased worker after occupational exposure. *Int Arch Occup Environ Health, 72(3)*,169–173.

Barregard, L., Sallsten, G., Schutz, A., Attewell, R., Skerfving, S., Jarvholm, B. (1992). Kinetics of mercury in blood and urine after brief occupational exposure. *Arch Environ Health, 47(3)*, 176–184.

Baughman, T. A. (2006). Elemental mercury spills. *Environ Health Perspect, 114(2)*, 147–152.

Bellinger, D. C., Trachtenberg, F., Barregard, L., Tavares, M., Cernichiari, E. & Daniel, D., et al. (2006). Neuropsychological and renal effects of dental amalgam in children: a randomized clinical trial. *JAMA, 295(15)*, 1775–1783.

Bronstein, A. C., Spyker, D. A., Cantilena, L. R., Jr., Green, J., Rumack, B. H. & Heard, S. E. (2007). 2006 annual report of the American Association of Poison Control Centers' National Poison Data System (NPDS). *Clin Toxicol (Phila), 45(8),* 815–917.

Burgess, J. L. (2007). Editorial on "exposure assessment of a mercury spill in a Nevada school—2004." *Clin Toxicol (Phila), 45(4)*, 43 1.

Caravati, E. M., Erdman, A. R., Christianson, G., Nelson, L. S., Woolf, A. D., Booze, L. L., et al. (2008). Elemental mercury exposure: An evidence-based consensus guideline for out-of-hospital management. *Clin Toxicol (Phila), 46(1)*, 1–21.

Carpi, A. & Chen, Y. F. (2001). Gaseous elemental mercury as an indoor air pollutant. *Environ Sci Technol, 35(21),* 4170–4173.

[CDC].Centers for Disease Control and Prevention. (2005a). Measuring exposure to an elemental mercury spill--Dakota County, Minnesota, 2004. *MMWR, 54(6)*, 146–149.

[CDC].Centers for Disease Control and Prevention. (2005b). Mercury exposure--Kentucky, 2004. *MMWR, 54(32)*, 797–799.

[CDC] Centers for Disease Control and Prevention. (2005c). Third national report on human exposure to environmental chemicals. Available from: http://www.cdc.gov/exposurereport/pdf/thirdreport.pdf [accessed 20 March 2008].

[CDC] Centers for Disease Control and Prevention. (2007). National Health and Nutrition Examination Survey. Available from: *http://www.cdc. gov/nchs/nhanes.htm* [accessed 28 January 2008].

Cherry, D., Lowry, L., Velez, L., Cotrell, C., Keyes, DC. (2002). Elemental mercury poisoning in a family of seven. *Fam Community Health, 24(4),* 1–8.

Chrysochoou, C., Rutishauser, C., Rauber-Luthy, C., Neuhaus, T., Boltshauser, E. & SupertiFurga, A. (2003). An 11-month-old boy with psychomotor regression and auto-aggressive behavior. *Eur J Pediatr, 162(7-8),* 559–561.

Cianciola, M. E., Echeverria, D., Martin, M. D., Aposian, H. V. & Woods, J. S. (1997). Epidemiologic assessment of measures used to indicate low-level exposure to mercury vapor (Hg). *J Toxicol Environ Health, 52(1)*, 19–33.

Clarkson, T. W. (2002). The three modern faces of mercury. *Environ Health Perspect 110 Suppl, 1*, 11–23.

[CNN] *CNN.com*. (2003). D.C. school to reopen after mercury spill. Available from: *http://www.cnn.com/2003/EDUCATION/11/04/mercury.spill. school.ap/*. [accessed 26 June 2008].

Davis, J. A. & Runkle, K. D. (2004). Reducing the risk of chemical exposures in schools. *J Environ Health, 67(5),* 9–13.

DeRouen, T. A., Martin, M. D., Leroux, B. G., Townes, B. D., Woods, J. S. & Leitao, J. et al. (2006). Neurobehavioral effects of dental amalgam in children: a randomized clinical trial. *JAMA, 295*(15),1784–1792.

[DHHS] U.S. Department of Health and Human Services. (2000). Healthy People 2010. Chapter 8: Environmental health section 8.25e. Available from: *http://www.healthypeople.gov/Document/HTML/ Volume1/08 Environmental.htm#_Toc4* 90564716 [accessed 25 September 2008].

[EPA] U.S. Environmental Protection Agency. (2002). Task force on ritualistic uses of mercury report. Available from: *http://www.epa. gov/superfund/community/pdfs/mercury.pdf* [accessed 26 June 2008].

Garetano, G., Stern, A. H., Robson, M. & Gochfeld, M. (2008). Mercury vapor in residential building common areas in communities where mercury is used for cultural purposes versus a reference community. *Sci Total Environ, 397(1-3),* 131–139.

Gattineni, J., Weiser, S., Becker, A. M. & Baum, M. (2007). Mercury intoxication: Lack of correlation between symptoms and levels. *Clin Pediatr (Phila), 46(9),* 844–846.

Goldstein A. (2000). *District joins effort to liquidate mercury*. Washington Post. September 27, Sect. B:2.

Gordon, A. T. (2004). Short-term elemental mercury exposures at three Arizona schools: Public health lessons learned. *J Toxicol Clin Toxicol, 42(2),* 179–187.

Hryhorczuk, D., Persky, V., Piorkowski, J., Davis, J., Moomey, C. M. & Krantz, A. et al. (2006). Residential mercury spills from gas regulators. *Environ Health Perspect, 114(6),* 848–852.

Hudson, P. J., Vogt, R. L., Brondum, J., Witherell, L., Myers, G., Paschal, D. C. (1987). Elemental mercury exposure among children of thermometer plant workers. *Pediatrics, 79(6),* 935–938.

Hursh, J. B., Cherian, M. G., Clarkson, T. W., Vostal, J. J. & Mallie, R. V. (1976). Clearance of mercury (HG-197, HG-203) vapor inhaled by human subjects. *Arch Environ Health, 31(6),* 302–309.

Hursh, J. B., Clarkson, T. W., Miles, E. F. & Goldsmith, L. A. (1989). Percutaneous absorption of mercury vapor by man. *Arch Environ Health, 44(2),* 120–127.

[IMERC] Interstate Mercury Education and Reduction Clearinghouse. (2008). 11 percent reduction in mercury use in products in the U.S. from 2001 to 2004, according to IMERC/NEWMOA report. Available from: http://www.newmoa.org/prevention/mercury/imerc/factsheets/mercuryinpr oducts_pressre lease.doc [accessed 8 July 2008].

Johnson, C. (1999). Elemental mercury use in religious and ritualistic practices in Latin American and Caribbean communities in New York. *Popul Environ, 20(5)*, 443–453.

Johnson, C. L. (2004). Mercury in the environment: Sources, toxicities, and prevention of exposure. *Pediatr Ann, 33(7)*, 437–442.

Jonsson, F., Sandborgh-Englund, G. & Johanson, G. (1999). A compartmental model for the kinetics of mercury vapor in humans. *Toxicol Appl Pharmacol, 155(2)*, 161–168.

[JSI] John Snow Inc. (2003). Ritual use of mercury (azogue) assessment and education project. Available from: http://www.jsi.com/Managed/Docs/ Publications/EnviroHealth/MercuryAssessment_Report.pdf [accessed 11 February 2008].

Kingman, A., Albertini, T. & Brown, L. J. (1998). Mercury concentrations in urine and whole blood associated with amalgam exposure in a U.S. military population. *J Dent Res, 77(3)*, 46 1–47 1.

Legislative-Council, State of Michigan. (2001). The revised school code (EXCERPT) Act 451 of 1976. Available from: *http://www. legislature.mi.gov/(S(ua3api45jdawkf453cwmxw45))/mileg.aspx?page=ge tO* bject&objectName=mcl-380-1274b [accessed 13 March 2008].

Link, B., Gabrio, T., Piechotowski, I., Zollner, I. & Schwenk, M. (2007). Baden-Wuerttemberg environmental health survey (BW-EHS) from 1996 to 2003: Toxic metals in blood and urine of children. *Int J Hyg Environ Health, 210(3-4)*, 357–371.

Lowry, L. K., Rountree, P. P., Levin, J. L., Collins, S. & Anger, W. K. (1999). The Texarkana mercury incident. *Tex Med, 95(10)*, 65–70.

[MDEQ] Michigan Department of Environmental Quality. (2007). Mercury P2. Available from: http://www.michigan.gov/deq/0,1607,7-135-3307_29693_4175---,00.html [accessed 10 December 2007].

[MPCA] Minnesota Pollution Control Agency. (2006). Minnesota's mercury initiative. Available from: http://proteus.pca.state.mn.us/air/ mercury-mn.html#initiative [accessed 10 December 2007].

Newby, A. C., Riley, D. M. & Leal-Almeraz, T. O. (2006). Mercury use and exposure among Santeria practitioners: Religious versus folk practice in northern New Jersey, USA. *Ethn Health, 11(3)*, 287–306.

[NIOSH] National Institute for Occupational Safety and Health. (1995). Report to congress on workers' home contamination study conducted under the Workers' Family Protection Act (29 U.S.C. 671a). Available from: http://www.cdc.gov/niosh/contamin.html [accessed 22 February 2008].

[NIOSH] National Institute for Occupational Safety and Health. (2006). School chemistry laboratory safety guide. Available from: http://wwwn.cdc.gov/pubs/niosh.aspx [accessed 28 February 2008].

[NJDEP] New Jersey Department of Environmental Protection. (2008). Decision document final remedial selection report. Accutherm, INC. Site Franklin Township, Gloucester County, New Jersey. Available from:http://www.state.nj.us/dep/srp/community/sites/accutherm/accuther m_dd.pdf [accessed 15 September 2008].

Orloff, K. G., Ulirsch, G., Wilder, L., Block, A., Fagliano, J. & Pasqualo, J. (1997). Human exposure to elemental mercury in a contaminated residential building. *Arch Environ Health, 52(3)*, 169–172.

Ozuah, P. O., Lesser, M. S., Woods, J. S., Choi, H. & Markowitz, M. (2003). Mercury exposure in an urban pediatric population. *Ambul Pediatr, 3(1)*, 24–26.

Putman, J. & Madden, R. (1972). Quicksilver and slow death. National Geographic Magazine: 506–527.

Rennie, A. C., McGregor-Schuerman, M., Dale, I. M., Robinson, C. & McWilliam, R. (1999). Mercury poisoning after spillage at home from a sphygmomanometer on loan from hospital. *BMJ, 319*(7206), 366–367.

Riley, D. M., Newby, C. A., Leal-Almeraz, T. O. & Thomas, V. M. (2001). Assessing elemental mercury vapor exposure from cultural and religious practices. *Environ Health Perspect, 109(8),* 779–784.

Roels, H. A., Boeckx, M., Ceulemans, E. & Lauwerys, R. R. (1991). Urinary excretion of mercury after occupational exposure to mercury vapor and influence of the chelating agent meso2,3-dimercaptosuccinic acid (DMSA). *Br J Ind Med, 48(4),* 247–253.

Rogers, H. S., Jeffery, N., Kieszak, S., Fritz, P., Spliethoff, H. & Palmer, C. D. et al. (2008). Mercury exposure in young children living in New York City. *J Urban Health, 85(1)*, 39–51.

Rogers, H. S., McCullough, J., Kieszak, S., Caldwell, K. L., Jones, R. L., Rubin, C. (2007). Exposure assessment of young children living in Chicago communities with historic reports of ritualistic use of mercury. *Clin Toxicol (Phila), 45(3),* 240–247.

Rytuba, J. J. (2000). Mercury mine drainage and processes that control its environmental impact. *Sci Total Environ. 260(1-3)*, 57–71.

Sandborgh-Englund, G., Elinder, C. G., Johanson, G., Lind, B. Skare, I. & Ekstrand, J. (1998). The absorption, blood levels, and excretion of mercury after a single dose of mercury vapor in humans. *Toxicol Appl Pharmacol, 150(1),* 146–153.

[SHP] Sustainable Hospitals Project. (2003). Mercury spills – How much do they cost? Available from: *http://www.sustainablehospitals. org/PDF/ IP_spills_cost.pdf* [accessed 9 September 2009].

Smart, E. R. (1986). Mercury vapor levels in a domestic environment following breakage of a clinical thermometer. *Sci Total Environ, 57*, 99–103.

Solis, M. T., Yuen, E., Cortez, P. S. & Goebel, P. J. (2000). Family poisoned by mercury vapor inhalation. *Am J Emerg Med, 18(5),* 599–602.

Taueg, C., Sanfilippo, D. J., Rowens, B., Szejda, J. & Hesse, J. L. (1992). Acute and chronic poisoning from residential exposures to elemental mercury--Michigan, 1989-1990. *J Toxicol Clin Toxicol, 30(1)*, 63–67.

Tominack, R., Weber, J., Blume, C., Madhok, M., Murphy, T. & Thompson, M., et al. (2002). Elemental mercury as an attractive nuisance: Multiple exposures from a pilfered school supply with severe consequences. *Pediatr Emerg Care, 18(2)*, 97–100.

Tunnessen, W. W., Jr., McMahon, K. J. & Baser, M. (1987). Acrodynia: Exposure to mercury from fluorescent light bulbs. *Pediatrics, 79(5),* 786–789.

von Muhlendahl, K. E. (1990). Intoxication from mercury spilled on carpets. *Lancet, 336(8730),* 1578.

Warkany J. (1966). Acrodynia--postmortem of a disease. *Am J Dis Child 1, 12(2),* 147–156

Wendroff, A. P. (2005). Magico-religious mercury use in Caribbean and Latino Communities: Pollution, persistence, and politics. *Environ Pract, 7*, 87–96.

[WHO] World Health Organization. (1991). Environmental health criteria 118: Inorganic mercury. Available from: *http://www.inchem.org /documents/ehc/ehc/ehc118.htm* [accessed 6 December 2007].

[WHO] World Health Organization. (2003). Concise international chemical assessment document 50—Elemental mercury and inorganic mercury compounds: Human health aspects. Geneva, Switzerland: Inter-Organization Programme for the Sound Management of Chemicals, International Program on Chemical Safety. Available from:

http://www.who.int/ipcs/publications/cicad/en/cicad50.pdf [accessed 11 January 2008].

Wossmann, W., Kohl, M., Gruning, G. & Bucsky, P. (1999). Mercury intoxication presenting with hypertension and tachycardia. *Arch Dis Child, 80(6)*, 556–557.

Zayas, L. H. & Ozuah, P. O. (1996). Mercury use in Espiritismo: A survey of botanicas. *Am J Public Health, 86(1)*, 111–112.

12. APPENDIX

Table 1. Geometric Means, Selected Percentiles, and the Corresponding 95% Confidence Intervals (CI) for Urine Mercury Concentrations (μg/L) for Children Sampled as Part of the National Health and Nutrition Examination Survey

Year Survey Conducted	Age Group in Years	Sample Size	Geometric Mean (95% CI)	Selected Percentile (95% CI)			
				50th	75th	90th	95th
2003–2004	6–11	286	0.254	0.190	0.430	1.14	1.96
			(0.213–0.304)	(0.160–0.230)	(0.330–0.560)	(0.610–1.61)	(1.13–2.97)
2003–2004	12–19	722	0.358	0.320	0.700	1.59	2.83
			(0.313–0.408)	(0.270–0.360)	(0.530–0.840)	(1.13–2.52)	(1.88–3.66)

Table 2. Federal, State, and Regional Programs that Capture Information on Releases of Hazardous Substances

Information Sources	Database	Internet URL
Federal Agencies		
• Agency for Toxic Substances and Disease Registry	• Health Consultations • Emergency Response • Hazardous Substances Emergency Events Surveillance	• www.atsdr.cdc.gov/HS/HSEES
• Centers for Disease Control and Prevention	• Clinical Information Service	• www.emergency.cdc.gov/coca/800cdcinfo. asp
• U.S. Coast Guard	• National Response Center Database	• www.nrc.uscg.mil/nrcback.html
• U.S. Environmental Protection Agency	• Superfund Information System • National Priorities List	• www.epa.gov/superfund/sites/siteinfo.htm • www.epa.gov/superfund/sites/query/advqu ery.htm
• National Institute for Occupational Safety and Health	• Report to Congress on Workers' Home Contamination Study Conducted Under the Workers' Family Protection Act (29 U.S.C. 671a)	• http://www.cdc.gov/niosh/contamin.html
Other Recognized Public Health Entities		
• American Association of Poison Control Centers	• National Poison Data System	• www.aapcc.org/dnn/NPDS/tabid/65/Defa ult.aspx
• Association of Occupational and Environmental Clinics	• Pediatric Environmental Health Specialty Units	• www.aoec.org/PEHSU.htm

Table 3. Overview of the Agency for Toxic Substances and Disease Registry (ATSDR) Health Consultations Involving U.S. Children Exposed to Elemental Mercury (Hg): Documented Between 2002–2007[*] (N=26)

Year Exposure Reported / Title of Health Consultation	State	Location	Estimated Hg Released ml	Max Hg in Air µ g/m[+]	Urine Hg Level µg/L	Blood Hg µg/L	Source of Mercury Exposure	URL
2002								
Hayes Middle School	MI	School	-	2	-	3	Mishap during science class demonstration	http://www.atsdr.cdc.gov/HAC/pha/hayes/hms_p1.html
Hg Spill Assist in Watervliet	MI	Home	-	5	10	-	Broken thermostat	http://www.atsdr.cdc.gov/HAC/pha/watervliet/msa_p1.html
Sarasota Residential Mercury Spill	FL	Home	237–296	43	4–5	-	Hg found at roadside and taken home	http://www.atsdr.cdc.gov/hac/pha/sarasotamercury/srm_p1.htm l#sum
Princeton Avenue Mercury Spill	MI	Home	167	4	-	-	Unknown source of Hg in furnace	None available
Spectrum Home Care Hg Spill Event	MI	Home	-	24	ND	-	12 broken thermometers	http://www.michigan.gov/documents/Spectrum_Home_Care_(thermometer)_102582_7.pdf
2003								
Mobile Medical Hg Spill	FL	Medical	-	10	-	ND	Leaking blood pressure calibration device	http://www.atsdr.cdc.gov/HAC/pha/MMIMercurySpill081103/MMIMercurySpill081103HC.pdf

Table 3. (Continued)

Year Exposure Reported Title of Health Consultation	State	Location	Estimated Hg Released ml	Max Hg in Air μg/m³	Urine Hg Level μg/L	Blood Hg μg/L	Source of Mercury Exposure	URL
Eastern Clinic Hg Spill	MI	Medical	-	42	-	-	Broken sphygmomanometer	http://www.atsdr.cdc.gov/HAC/pha/EasternClinic110503-MI/EasternClinic_HC110503.pdf
Durand Hg Incident	MI	Home	296–355	-	-	ND	Children stole vials of Hg from junkyard	http://www.atsdr.cdc.gov/HAC/PHA/durandmercury/dmi_toc.html
Rosemore Middle School	OH	School Home	25	58	-	-	Child brought vial of Hg from home to school	http://www.atsdr.cdc.gov/HAC/pha/rosemore/rms_p1.html
Hg Exposures from 3M Tartan Brand Floors	OH	School	-	2	-	-	Hg off gassing from Hg catalyst in gym floor	http://www.atsdr.cdc.gov/HAC/pha/westerville/wes_p1.html
2004								
Locust Grove Hg Response Site	GA	Home	12	36	-	-	Children stole and dismantled 2 sphygmomanometers and took Hg home	http://www.atsdr.cdc.gov/HAC/pha/locustgrove/loc_toc.html
St. Louis Residential Hg Spill	MI	Home	-	0.1	-	-	Broken thermometer	http://www.atsdr.cdc.gov/HAC/pha/StLouisResidentialMercury050604-MI/StLouisResidentialMercuryHC050604.pdf

Table 3. (Continued)

Year Exposure Reported Title of Health Consultation	State	Location	Estimated Hg Released ml	Max Hg in Air μ g/m³‡	Urine Hg Level μg/L	Blood Hg μg/L	Source of Mercury Exposure	URL
Benton Harbor Residential Hg Spill	MI	Home	9–16	>92	-	29	Broken sphygmomanometer	http://www.atsdr.cdc.gov/HAC/ph a/BentonHarbor102604HC-MI/BentonHarbor102604HC-MI.pdf
Charlotte Middle School Hg Incident	MI	School	-	8	-	-	3 10-inch thermometers broken during science class	http://www.atsdr.cdc.gov/HAC/ph a/CharlotteMiddleSchoolMercury0 72104-MI/CharlotteMidSchool072104-MI.pdf
Mid-Michigan Hg Floor	MI	School	-	0.05	-	-	Hg off-gassing from Hg catalyst in gym floor	http://www.atsdr.cdc.gov/HAC/pha/Mid-MichiganMercuryFloor050604-MI/Mid-MichiganMercuryFloorHC 050604.pdf
Rosemont Woods Hg Incident	MN	13 Homes1 Car	700	-	< 10†	< 4 to 13$	Children stole Hg from industrial site and dispersed it among other children	http://www.atsdr.cdc.gov/HAC/ph a/Rosemount%620Woods%620 Mercury%20Incident/Rosemount WoodsHC071305.pdf
Luxemburg Single Residence Mercury Spill	WI	Home	-	0.6	-	-	Hg spilt from broken thermostat switch	http://www.atsdr.cdc.gov/HAC/ph a/Luxemburg022305-WI/Luxemburg022305-WI.pdf

Table 3. (Continued)

Year Exposure Reported Title of Health Consultation	State	Location	Estimated Hg Released ml	Max Hg in Air μ g/m³	Urine Hg Level μg/L	Blood Hg μg/L	Source of Mercury Exposure	URL
Stoughton High School Mercury Spill	WI	School	59	22	6	-	Accidental glass manometer spilt Hg	http://www.atsdr.cdc.gov/HAC/pha/stoughtonhs/shs_p1.html#sum
2005								
El Camino Middle School Hg Spill	CA	School	-	>20	-	-	Student brought 35 mm film canister of Hg to school and played with it	http://www.atsdr.cdc.gov/HAC/pha/El%20Camino%20Mercury%20Spill/ElCaminoMercurySpillHC10-04-05.pdf
Hg Contamination in Indoor Air	KY	Home	-	50	-	-	Multiple Hg vials stored in home may have leaked or been played with	http://www.atsdr.cdc.gov/HAC/pha/StateofKYMercury031505-KY/StateofKYMercury031505-KY.pdf
2006								
Kingsford Middle School	MI	School	-	< 3	-	-	Teacher poured Hg on desk to show students the physical properties of Hg. Hg then recaptured and brought home.	http://michigan.gov/documents/mdch/Kingsford_Middle_School_spill_225681_7.pdf
Petersburg Hg Site	MI	Home	-	11	ND	< 4	Unknown	http://www.michigan.gov/documents/mdch/Petersburg_HC_home_workshop_225964_7.pdf

Table 3. (Continued)

Year Exposure Reported Title of Health Consultation	State	Location	Estimated Hg Released ml	Max Hg in Air μ g/m³‡	Urine Hg Level μg/L†	Blood Hg μg/L$	Source of Mercury Exposure	URL
Ontonagon High School Hg Release	MI	School	33	9	-	-	Accidental spill at school	http://www.atsdr.cdc.gov/HAC/pha/OntonagonHighSchoolMercurzRelease/OntonoganHighSchoolHC033007.pdf
Hg-Containing Polyurethane Floors in Minnesota Schools	MN	School	-	3	-	-	Hg off-gassing from Hg catalyst in gym floor	http://www.atsdr.cdc.gov/HAC/pha/MercuryVaporReleaseAthleticPolymerFloors/MercuryVaporRelease-FloorsHC092806.pdf
Kiddie Kollge	NJ	Daycare	-	13	Max of 18†	-	Building formerly used to manufacture mercury thermometers	http://www.atsdr.cdc.gov/HAC/pha/KiddieKollege/KiddieKollegeHC061307.pdf
Salem-Keizer School District 3M Flooring	OR	School	-	2	-	-	Hg off-gassing from Hg catalyst in gym floor	http://www.atsdr.cdc.gov/HAC/pha/SalemKeizerSchoolDistrict/Salem-KeizerSchoolHC071206.pdf

ª Health Consults were queried based on completion date (2002 – 2007). However, the actual exposure may have taken place prior to the year the Health Consult was finalized.

† μg/g creatinine

‡ If more than one vapor Hg level was given, the reported level reflected the maximum level in a breathing zone or living space. ATSDR Minimal Risk Level for chronic mercury inhalation is 0.2 μg/m 3.

$ Blood mercury results reported for 2 days after exposure.

ND = No level detected

Table 4. Characteristics of Hazardous Substances Emergency Events Surveillance (HSEES)-Reported Mercury Events: 2002–2006*

	N	%
Mercury Events	843	100
Events Affecting Children	409	49
State Reporting Event		
Reporting all 5 years		
Colorado	5	1
Louisiana	8	2
Minnesota	56	14
New Jersey	73	18
New York	129	32
North Carolina	5	1
Oregon	4	1
Texas	6	2
Utah	19	5
Washington	7	2
Wisconsin	32	8
Reporting 4 years		
Missouri	39	10
Reporting 2 years		
Alabama	0	0
Florida	7	2
Michigan	16	4
Mississippi		

	N	%
Type of Release		
Spill Only	360	88
Volatilization	6	2
Spill and Volatilization	40	10
Fire	1	<1
Not reported	2	<1
Location of Event		
Private household	307	75
School†	98	24
Other	4	1
Contributing Cause of Event		
Equipment failure	27	7
Human error	357	87
Intentional or illegal release	18	4
Unknown	7	2

* Percentages may total beyond 100% due to rounding error.

† Includes private property other than a home (3) and restaurant (1).

Table 5. Mercury Events Reported to the National Response Center by Year[*]: 2002–2007

Year Reported	Number of Hg Events	Number of Events in Which Children were Potentially Exposed
2002	164	14
2003	98	13
2004	111	22
2005	158	20
2006	142	24
2007	152	20
Total (2002–2007)	825	113

* The actual exposure may have taken place prior to the year the spill event was reported.

Table 6. Mercury Events Reported to the National Response Center that Potentially Exposed Children by Location: 2002–2007 (N= 113)

Category	Number[*]
School	50
Home	5
Medical facility or clinic	1
Other location[†]	14
Location not reported	45

* Exposure locations are not mutually exclusive; therefore, the number of locations does not total the number of reported events (N=113). In addition, location is likely biased by the selection criteria of including all exposure events at schools or daycare facilities.

† Category includes street addresses when the specific location (i.e., school or home) could not be determined.

Table 7. Number and Percentage of Non-Thermometer-Related Calls to the American Association of Poison Control Centers by Mercury Subclassifications: 2002–2006[*]

Year	Mercury Type	Total Calls Received # (%)	Calls Regarding Children ~ 19 Years of Age # (%)	Calls Regarding Children as Percentage of Total Calls Received
2002				
	Mercury	3,754 (100)	1,540 (100)	41
	Elemental[†]	3,577 (95)	1,495 (97)	42
	Inorganic	34 (1)	11 (1)	32
	Other[‡]	143 (4)	34 (2)	24
2003				
	Mercury	3,292 (100)	1,584 (100)	48
	Elemental[†]	3,003 (91)	1,494 (94)	50
	Inorganic	38 (1)	8 (1)	21
	Other[‡]	251 (8)	82 (5)	33
2004				
	Mercury	3,023 (100)	1,440 (100)	48
	Elemental[†]	2,739 (91)	1,350 (94)	49
	Inorganic	53 (2)	16 (1)	30
	Other[‡]	231 (8)	74 (5)	32
2005				
	Mercury	3,051 (100)	1,213 (100)	40
	Elemental[†]	2,639 (86)	1,109 (91)	42
	Inorganic	54 (2)	8 (1)	15
	Other[‡]	358 (12)	96 (8)	27
2006				
	Mercury	2,619 (100)	999 (100)	38
	Elemental[†]	2,420 (92)	948 (95)	39
	Inorganic	26 (1)	7 (1)	27
	Other[‡]	173 (7)	44 (4)	25
Total for all 5 years (2002– 2006)	Mercury	15,739 (100)	6,776 (100)	43
	Elemental[†]	14,378 (91)	6,396 (94)	44
	Inorganic	205 (1)	50 (1)	24
	Other[‡]	1,156 (7)	330 (5)	29

[*] Percent totals may not equal zero due to rounding errors.

[†] Does not include amalgams or thermometers

[‡] Includes amalgams, organic mercury, "unknown," etc.

Table 8. Number and Percentage of Calls to the American Association of Poison Control Centers Regarding Human Exposure to Mercury Thermometers: 2002–2006

Year	Thermometer Type	Total Calls Received	Calls Regarding Children ≤ 19 Years of Age	Children as Percentage of Total Calls Received
2002	General formulation	12,466	8,450	68
	Basal	650	471	72
	Hi low	668	449	67
	Oral fever	625	381	61
	Baby rectal	492	346	70
	Yellow back glass	10	7	70
	Mercury metal	6	4	67
2003	General formulation	10,136	7,137	70
	Basal	467	327	70
	Hi low	371	241	65
	Oral fever	509	350	69
	Baby rectal	307	213	69
	Yellow back glass	7	5	71
	Mercury metal	2	1	50
2004	General formulation	6,432	4,486	70
	Basal	325	210	65
	Hi low	302	189	63
	Oral fever	374	259	69
	Baby rectal	176	132	75
	Yellow back glass	3	3	100
	Mercury metal	3	1	33
2005	General formulation	5,472	3,650	67
	Basal	314	194	62
	Hi low	183	126	69
	Oral fever	364	259	71
	Baby rectal	157	103	66
	Yellow back glass	2	0	0
	Mercury metal	2	1	50

Table 8. (Continued)

Year	Thermometer Type	Total Calls Received	Calls Regarding Children ≤19 Years of Age	Children as Percentage of Total Calls Received
2006	General formulation	3,538	2,349	66
	Basal	243	153	63
	Hi low	171	96	56
	Oral fever	318	218	69
	Baby rectal	127	78	61
	Yellow back glass	9	2	22
	Mercury metal	1	0	0
	General formulation	38,044	26,072	69
Total for all 5 years (2002–2006)	Basal	1,999	1,355	68
	Hi low	1,695	1,101	65
	Oral fever	2,190	1,467	67
	Baby rectal	1,259	872	69
	Yellow back glass	31	17	55
	Mercury metal	14	7	50

Table 9. Peer-Reviewed Literature Reporting Elemental Mercury (Hg) Exposures Involving U.S. Children: Published Between 2002–2007

Year of Exposure	Exposure Location	Amt. of Hg Spilled ml	# of Children Exposed	Age	Exposure Duration	Source of Mercury Exposure	Vapor Mercury Levels[6] μ g/m^3	Hg in Blood μ g/L	Hg in Urine μ g/L	Reported Symptoms[1]	References
NR*	Home Car School	180–480	19	2–18	1 month	Youth stole Hg from school. Gave Hg to other youth who dispersed Hg at home and school.	1,764 in 1 home 143 in 1 car< 3at school	-	≤428	Back, leg, joint, stomach, muscle pain, painful urination, constipation, night sweats, peeling feet and fingers, red hands, rash, poor sleep, edema, desquamation of palms, groin pain, constipation, impotence, Guillain-Barre syndrome, headaches, high blood pressure, insomnia, acrodynia	Tominack 2002
NR	Home	unknown	1	8	4 months	Hg was found dripping from the kitchen	6.5	-	12	Pain and decreased motor strength in both lower	Gattineni 2007

Table 9. (Continued)

Year of Exposure	Exposure Location	Amt. of Hg Spilled ml	# of Children Exposed	Age	Exposure Duration	Source of Mercury Exposure	Vapor Mercury Levels[6] μ g/m³	Hg in Blood μ g/L	Hg in Urine μ g/L	Reported Symptoms[1]	References
						stove vent				extremities, burning sensation in hands and feet, headache, dizziness, nausea, constipation, suppressed appetite, waddling gait, and irritability	
1993	Home	33	4	10–17	1 month	Youth stole Hg from school. Youth and siblings played with Hg at home and applied to skin.	110–140 4 months after initial exposure	-	586–1,348	Unable to walk and stand, seizures, rash, nausea, vomiting, fever, cough, thrombocytopenia platelets, elanotic stool with bright red blood, fever, and respiratory arrest	Baughman 2006
1994	Home	33	Several children	NR	2 hours	Children played with and broke Hg-containing medical device.	Up to 30	-	-	NR	

Table 9. (Continued)

Year[5] of Exposure	Exposure Location	Amt. of Hg Spilled ml	# of Children Exposed	Age	Exposure Duration	Source of Mercury Exposure	Vapor Mercury Levels[6] in µg/m³	Hg in Blood in µg/L	Hg in Urine in µg/L	Reported Symptoms[1]	References
1998	School Home	30	182	Adolescent	Minutes to 3 days	Youth stole Hg from school science room. Sold to other students. Some took Hg home.	< 5 – 702 at school			Headache, itching, sore throat, coughing, abdomi-nal pain, nausea, dizzy, runny nose, diarrhea, shortness of breath, vomiting, fever, metallic taste, chest pain	
1998	School Home	30	74	11–18 yrs	≤ 16 days	Youth stole Hg from school science room. Gave Hg to other students. Some took Hg home.	< 5 at school	20–32	≤ 0.20	NR	Gordon 2005
1998	School Home	unknown	18	NR	NR	NR	11–30			NR	
2000 and earlier	1,363 Homes	per house ≤ 10	NR	NR	NR	Hg spilled during removal of gas regulator	27 – 78 in one home	16 for one child	10–263	Headaches, rash	Hryho-rczuk 2006

Table 9. (Continued)

Year of Exposure	Exposure Location	Amt. of Hg Spilled ml	# of Children Exposed	Age	Exposure Duration	Source of Mercury Exposure	Vapor Mercury Levels µ g/m³	Hg in Blood µ g/L	Hg in Urine µ g/L	Reported Symptoms	References
2000	Home	NR	5	3–16	≤ 9 months	Prior tenants of mobile home left container of Hg in closet. Container believed to be spilled on carpet.	NR	295	600–2,940 µg/24-hour sample	Weight loss, limping, ataxia, irritability, speech regression, tachycardia, hypertensive	Cherry 2002
2003	School Home	NR	1,000	Adolescent	NR	16-year-old student took Hg from chemistry lab. Hg spread around school and several homes	NR	NR	NR	NR	Johnson 2004 CNN 2003
2004	School School Bus	60	55	Adolescent	<12 hours	Youth stole Hg from school. Gave Hg to other youth who dispersed Hg at home and school. Hg played with on school bus and school.	>50	NR	Mean 0.36	Respiratory	Azziz-Baumgartner 2004

Table 9. (Continued)

Year of Exposure	Exposure Location	Amt. of Hg Spilled ml	# of Children Exposed	Age	Exposure Duration	Source of Mercury Exposure	Vapor Mercury Levels[6] μg/m³	Hg in Blood μg/L	Hg in Urine μg/L	Reported Symptoms[1]	References
2004	Outdoors Home	701	14	6–16 yrs	<2 hrs	Youth stole Hg from industrial site. Gave Hg to other youth and played with it.	0.06 to 50	<4 to 13	3–<10[2]	Cough, loss of appetite	CDC 2005b
2004	School Bus School Home	unknown	15 at school 6 at home	Adolescent	<1 day at school 15 months at home	Youth stole Hg from dental office and brought to school. Gave Hg to other youth and played with it.	5.3 to 36.6 School >50 home	32–72[3]	28–496	Rashes, headaches, tachycardia, hypertension, desquamation of soles and palms, diaphoresis, muscle pain, insomnia, vomiting, and behavioral and psychiatric changes	CDC 2005c

NR = Not Reported

[1] Not all children exposed had symptoms

[2] μg/g creatinine

[3] Includes adults

[4] μg/ml

[5] Year of exposure rather than publication year is presented; in some cases the exposure occurred several years prior to the publication.

[6] ATSDR Minimal Risk Level for chronic mercury inhalation is 0.2 μg/m³.

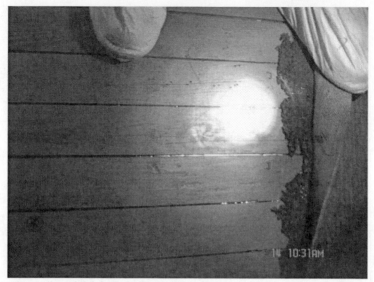

Photograph and additional information available from *http://www.epaosc.net/ site_profile.asp?site_id=3372* Accessed 27 February 2008

Figure 1a. Mercury Contamination in Floorboards of a Residential Home.

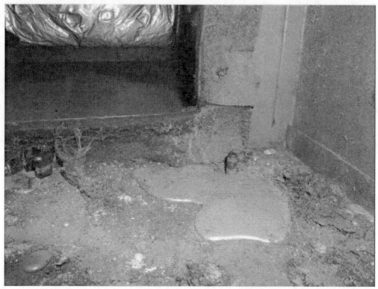

Photograph obtained from the Michigan Department of Community Health

Figure 1b. Mercury Contamination Near a Residential Furnace.

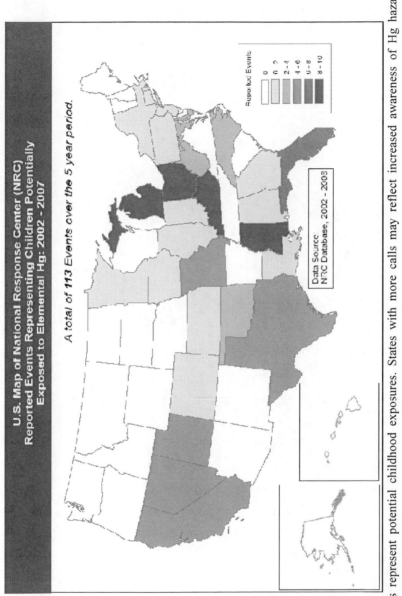

NRC events represent potential childhood exposures. States with more calls may reflect increased awareness of Hg hazards and subsequently increased reporting.

Figure 2. (Continued)

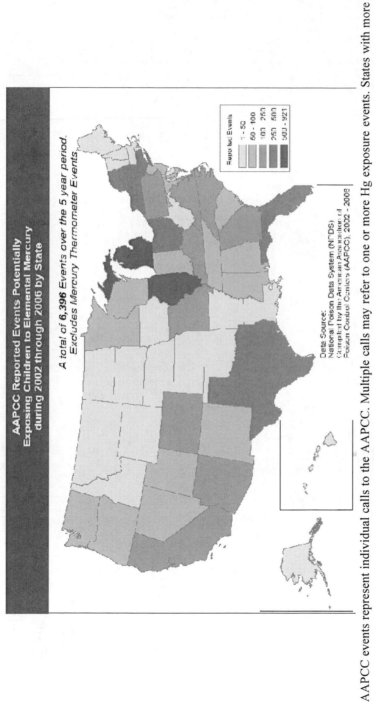

AAPCC events represent individual calls to the AAPCC. Multiple calls may refer to one or more Hg exposure events. States with more calls may reflect increased awareness of Hg hazards and subsequently increased reporting.

Figure 2. Maps of the United States Representing Mercury (Hg) Events Potentially Exposing Children to Elemental Hg as Reported by the National Response Center (NRC) and Elemental Hg Calls to the American Association of Poison Control Centers (AAPCC) by State.

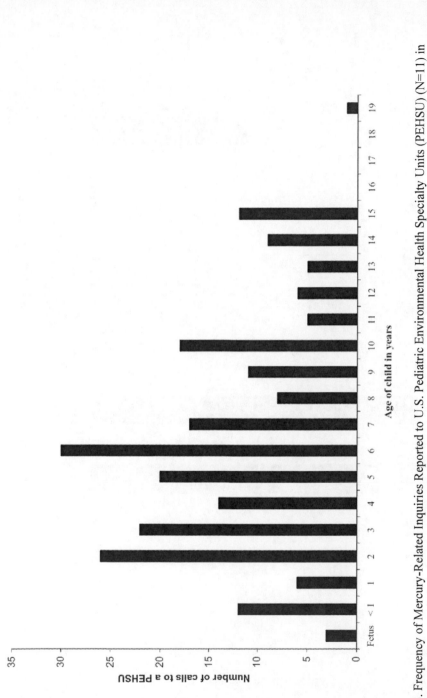

Figure 3. Frequency of Mercury-Related Inquiries Reported to U.S. Pediatric Environmental Health Specialty Units (PEHSU) (N=11) in Which the Age of the Child in Question was Known (N=225).

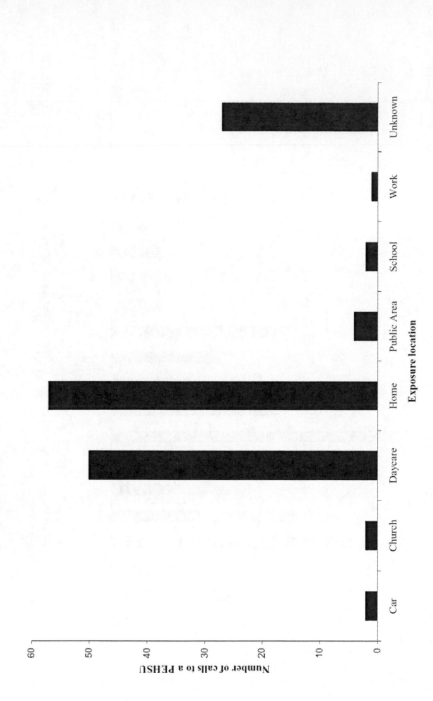

Figure 4. Frequency of Mercury-Related Inquires Reported to U.S. Pediatric Environmental Health Specialty Units (PEHSU) (N=11) by Exposure Location (N=145).

SUPPLEMENTAL MATERIAL

Initiatives That May Reduce Exposure Frequency

To further assess the extent of children's exposure to mercury from former industrial sites and other sources nationwide, the workgroup reviewed and described a number of ongoing initiatives and available resources that impact the occurrence and frequency of these events. This list is not intended to be an exhaustive list.

Ongoing Efforts to Reduce Exposure to Elemental Mercury

A number of federal and state-based initiatives affect the potential for childhood mercury exposures.

Federal Initiatives. Congress passed the Small Business Liability Relief and Brownfields Revitalization Act in 2002, setting up the funding of grants for brownfields activities administered by EPA. Brownfields are defined in the statute as "real property, the expansion, redevelopment, or reuse of which may be complicated by the presence or potential presence of a hazardous substance, pollutant, or contaminant." The EPA Brownfields program awards grants to state, tribal and local governments and not for profit organizations to assess and clean up eligible brownfields, including sites that may have been contaminated with mercury through industrial activity or illegal disposal (http://www.epa.gov/brownfields). States may oversee assessment and cleanup activities, where appropriate, to ensure the cleanup meets state standards."

Through its role in the brownfields initiative, ATSDR created a Brownfields/Land Reuse Steering Committee, composed of ATSDR, EPA, and state partners, to assess the impacts of redevelopment on public health. This effort includes the broader health impacts of revitalization and a sustainable environment.

In another federal initiative, ATSDR and state partners have created a workgroup to address concerns regarding mercury vapor release from floor covering. The intent of this group is to provide more detailed information on the environmental and human health concerns for staff and students who attend schools with polyurethane floors that contain a mercury catalyst. Local school authorities will use the information gathered to make informed risk management decisions and to provide parents and students with appropriate information on potential health risks.

Mercury is found in many schools, often in such equipment as thermometers and barometers. Accidental exposures to mercury due to equipment breakage or spills can have negative effects on children's health. Since mercury spills in schools are usually caused by improper storage or mishandling of mercury containing equipment, EPA actively encourages schools to prevent mercury spills by removing all mercury mercury-containing equipment. EPA's "Schools Chemical Cleanout Campaign" provides schools with information and tools to help them identify and remove mercury equipment and supplies. Extensive additional information for schools is available on EPA's website, http://epa.gov/mercury/schools.htm.

State Initiatives. A few states have passed laws that affect locating schools and redeveloping property for use as a school. Ten states have laws that prohibit locating a school on or near pollution sources, including mercury-contaminated sites. Six states require environmental assessments for any new school locations. However, the vast majority of states have yet to adopt such regulations.

To reduce the amount of mercury entering the waste stream and lessen the incidence of spills and exposures, some states have restricted the sale and disposal of mercury- containing products. For example, legislation was enacted (or proposed) regarding the sale or disposal of mercury-containing thermometers, thermostats, switches, relays, blood pressure devices, electronic appliances, batteries, and dental amalgams. Some legislation specifically targets the use of products containing mercury in schools or health care settings. EPA provides a table of mercury legislation, regulations, resolutions, and county/city ordinances by state on its Web site (*http://www.epa. gov/epawaste/hazard/tsd/mercury/laws.htm*). Currently, there are 45 states with mercury initiatives.

As an example of a specific state-based initiative, the Michigan Department of Environmental Quality has released a comprehensive strategy to eliminate the use and release of mercury. The details of this strategy are available at *http://www.michigan.gov/documents/deq/MDEQ_MSWG_FinalReportJan2008.pdf_222* 256 _7.pdf. This comprehensive plan addresses mercury releases to air, land, waste, and water and outlines Michigan's rules, regulations, policies, and monitoring activities. The Michigan Department of Community Health (MDCH) has also launched a mercury Web site (www.michigan.gov/mercury) to provide information to homeowners, schools, businesses, and responders. MDCH also joined with AAPCC, EPA, and local health departments to provide information to local communities on how to handle spills.

In addition to enacting legislation that prohibits the use of mercury and limits the availability of products containing mercury in schools, some states have developed initiatives to proactively educate teachers and students regarding the potential dangers of mercury exposures and to assist in school laboratory cleanouts. For example, the Illinois Department of Public Health (IDPH) has an interactive mercury education Web site (http://app.idph.state.il.us/envhealth/mercury/Default.htm) that includes curricula for teachers, information on handling spills in the classroom, and activities for children to learn how to avoid exposure. In addition, as part of a program to reduce the risks of chemical hazards in schools, including mercury, IDPH hosts 10 to 12 training workshops for teachers each year and has specifically targeted mercury hazards [Davis and Runkle 2004]. Not all state initiatives are this comprehensive.

Selected Resources with Information on Preventing Mercury Exposure

The following resources may help organizations or individuals who seek information on preventing mercury exposures, responding appropriately to environmental contamination, and evaluating and caring for exposed children. These resources are not intended to represent the universe of available and useful resources. Although these resources are generally useful, information from sources other than CDC/ATSDR was not formally reviewed and do not represent any CDC/ATSDR determination or policy.

General Information. The United Nations Environment Programme has established a Web site (http://www.chem.unep.ch/mercury/) to increase awareness of the health and environmental issues related to mercury. The Web site includes questions and answers, links to international mercury Web sites, and the reports of an international workgroup on mercury. Although it is not limited to elemental mercury, the site includes several useful resources and guidance on reducing mercury exposure.

Individuals who are interested in what products contain mercury may find the Interstate Mercury Education & Reduction Clearinghouse's (IMERC) Mercury-added Products database useful (www.newmoa.org/prevention /mercury/imerc/notification). This websites gives information on a wide variety of products that contain mercury.

An organization called Healthcare Without Harm maintains a Web site (http://www.noharm.org/us/mercury/alternatives) with recommendations on alternatives to mercury-containing products (e.g., digital thermometers) and on starting community grassroots efforts to reduce or eliminate mercury in communities.

The University of Wisconsin maintains a Web site (http://www.mercuryinschools.uwex.edu/) designed to reduce the impact of mercury spills in schools. It serves as a clearinghouse for information about mercury and related health concerns. This site includes lesson plans for teachers and links to resources to address mercury issues in the community.

The Maine Department of Environmental Protection released a report in 2008 titled, "Maine Compact Fluorescent Lamp Study." The report evaluated different cleanup methods for effectiveness. The report is available at: http://www.maine.gov/dep/rwm/homeowner/cflreport/cflreportwoapp.pdf

The CDC Clinical Information Service is a toll-free hotline (800.CDC.INFO or 800.232.4636) that is serviced 24 hours a day, 365 days a year. The service can rapidly disseminate CDC health-related materials and information (e.g., posters, pamphlets, CDROMs) to clinicians and the public.

In addition, the CDC and ATSDR Web sites contain numerous links online mercury information. The ATSDR Mercury Toxicological Profile (http://www.atsdr.cdc.gov/toxprofiles/tp46.html#bookmark01) is a peer-reviewed document that identifies and reviews the key literature regarding mercury's toxicological properties and adverse health effects. The indented audiences include health professionals at federal, state, and local levels; academicians; nonprofit/environmental groups, and interested members of the public.

ToxFAQs™ for Mercury (http://www.atsdr.cdc.gov/tfacts46.html) is a quick and easy fact sheet on mercury. Answers are provided to the most frequently asked questions about exposure to mercury. The intended audience is the lay community.

The ToxFAQs™ CABS for Mercury_(http://www.atsdr.cdc.gov/cabs/mercury/index.htm) provides current and relevant scientific information on mercury for public officials, business leaders, concerned citizens, and others to use in their work.

The ATSDR Pediatric Environmental Health Case Study in Environmental Medicine (CSEM) Appendix B_(http://www.atsdr.cdc.gov/csem/pediatric/appendixb.html) is a case study designed to increase the primary care provider's knowledge of mercury in the environment and to aid in the evaluation of potentially exposed pediatric patients.

Another link is to the joint ATSDR and EPA National Alert on metallic or elemental mercury exposures. The alert, titled "National Alert on Mercury: A

Warning about Continuing Patterns of Metallic Mercury Exposure," is available at (http://www.atsdr.cdc.gov/alerts/970626.html). The alert includes general information on mercury, cleanup procedures, and how to prevent exposures. The intended audiences are parents and educators.

EPA also provides a web portal to numerous EPA materials on mercury (http://www.epa.gov/mercury). The web site includes a link to information on how to clean up mercury spills (http://www.epa.gov/mercury/spills/index. htm). The guidance on the web site provides information on safely handling small mercury spills in homes (e.g., broken thermometers). The site also provides information regarding the proper disposal of mercury-containing products.

School-Based Information. EPA maintains a Web site titled "Schools and Mercury" (http://www.epa.gov/mercury/schools.htm). The purpose of this Web site is to provide information to enable school administrators and staff to effectively reduce the risk of mercury exposure in schools.

The National Institute of Environmental Health Sciences provides the following Web site for students: http://www.niehs.nih.gov/health/topics/ agents/lead/docs/ComparingTwoEnvironmentalE   vils.pdf. The Web site provides a lesson plan to teach students about mercury poisoning and compares and contrasts the health effects of mercury and lead. The information on these pages provides useful resources to parents, guardians, and caretakers of children.

In 2006, NIOSH published a guidance document on school chemistry laboratory safety [NIOSH 2006]. This document advocates the appropriate management of mercury in the classroom, which may help reduce or mitigate the many school-based mercury spills reported in the various databases.

End Notes

[1] The simple arithmetic mean is not suitable for representing "average" when observations are not normally distributed. The occurrence of a few high or low numbers could result in a perceived "average" that is not reflective of actual conditions. In such situations statisticians use the geometric mean as a more appropriate measure of central tendency.

In: Child Exposure to Elemental Mercury   ISBN: 978-1-61470-941-1
Editors: R. Rustoen and S. Ziegler   © 2012 Nova Science Publishers, Inc.

Chapter 2

MERCURY[*]

Centers for Disease Control and Prevention

Mercury is an element and a metal that is found in air, water, and soil. It exists in three forms that have different properties, usage, and toxicity. The three forms are called elemental (or metallic) mercury, inorganic mercury compounds, and organic mercury compounds.

Elemental mercury is liquid at room temperature. It is used in some thermometers, dental amalgams, fluorescent light bulbs, some electrical switches, mining, and some industrial processes. It is released into the air when coal and other fossil fuels are burned.

Inorganic mercury compounds are formed when mercury combines with other elements, such as sulfur or oxygen, to form compounds or salts. Inorganic mercury compounds can occur naturally in the environment. Inorganic mercury compounds are used in some industrial processes and in the making of other chemicals. Outside the United States, inorganic mercury salts have been used in cosmetic skin creams.

Organic mercury compounds are formed when mercury combines with carbon. Microscopic organisms in water and soil can convert elemental and

---

[*] This is an edited, reformatted and augmented version of a Centers for Disease Control and Prevention publication, dated November 2009.

inorganic mercury into an organic mercury compound, methylmercury, which accumulates in the food chain. Thimerosal and phenylmercuric acetate are other types of organic mercury compounds made in small amounts for use as preservatives.

HOW PEOPLE ARE EXPOSED TO MERCURY

Elemental mercury: People may be exposed when they breathe air containing elemental mercury vapors. Vapors may be present in such workplaces as dental offices, smelting operations, and locations where mercury has been spilled or released. In the body, elemental mercury can be converted to inorganic mercury.

Inorganic Mercury: People may be exposed if they work where inorganic mercury compounds are used.

Organic Mercury: People may be exposed when they eat fish or shellfish contaminated with methylmercury. Methylmercury can pass through the placenta, exposing the developing fetus.

HOW MERCURY AFFECTS PEOPLE'S HEALTH

Elemental mercury: The human health effects from exposure to low environmental levels of elemental mercury are unknown. Very high mercury vapor concentrations can quickly cause severe lung damage. At low vapor concentrations over a long time, neurological disturbances, memory problems, skin rash, and kidney abnormalities may occur.

Inorganic Mercury: When eaten in large amounts, some inorganic mercury compounds can be very irritating and corrosive to the digestive system. If repeatedly eaten or applied to the skin over long period of time, some inorganic mercury compounds can cause effects similar to what is seen with long term mercury vapor exposure, including neurological disturbances, memory problems, skin rash, and kidney abnormalities.

Organic Mercury: Large amounts of methylmercury eaten over weeks to months have caused damage to the nervous system. Infants born to women who were poisoned with methylmercury had developmental abnormalities and cerebral palsy.

LEVELS OF MERCURY IN THE U.S. POPULATION

In the *Fourth National Report on Human Exposure to Environmental Chemicals (Fourth Report),* CDC scientists measured total mercury in the blood of 8,373 participants aged one year and older who took part in the National Health and Nutrition Examination Survey (NHANES) during 2003–2004. Total blood mercury is mainly a measure of methyl mercury exposure. In the same 2003–2004 NHANES, CDC scientists measured mercury in the urine of 2,538 participants aged six years and older. Mercury in the urine is a measure of inorganic mercury exposure. By measuring mercury in blood and in urine, scientists can estimate the amount of mercury that has entered people's bodies.

- CDC scientists found measureable mercury in most of the participants. Both blood and urine mercury levels tend to increase with age.
- Defining safe levels of mercury in blood continues to be an active research area. In 2000, the National Research Council of the National Academy of Sciences determined that a level of 85 micrograms per liter (µg/L) in cord blood was associated with early neurodevelopmental effects. The lower 95% confidence limit of this estimate was 58 µg/L. All blood mercury levels for persons in this *Report* were less than 33 µg/L.
- Blood and urine mercury in the U.S. population were similar to levels seen in other developed countries.

Finding a measurable amount of mercury in blood or urine does not mean that levels of mercury cause an adverse health effect. Biomonitoring studies on levels of mercury provide physicians and public health officials with reference values so that they can determine whether people have been exposed to higher levels of mercury than are found in the general population. Biomonitoring data can also help scientists plan and conduct research about exposure and health effects.

For More Information

- Agency for Toxic Substances and Disease Registry
  A Warning about Continuing Patterns of Metallic Mercury Exposure
  http://www.atsdr.cdc.gov/alerts/970626.html
  ToxFAQs for Mercury
  http://www.atsdr.cdc.gov/cabs/mercury/index.html
- CDC Emergency Preparedness and Response
  Mercury
  http://emergency.cdc.gov/agent/mercury/
- Environmental Protection Agency
  Mercury: Basic Information
  http://www.epa.gov/mercury/about.htm
- Food and Drug Administration
  What You Need to Know About Mercury in Fish and Shellfish
  http://www.fda.gov/Food/FoodSafety/Product-
  SpecificInformation/Seafood/FoodbornePathogensContaminants/Met
  hylmercury/ucm1 15662 .htm

November 2009

The Centers for Disease Control and Prevention (CDC) protects people's health and safety by preventing and controlling diseases and injuries; enhances health decisions by providing credible information on critical health issues; and promotes healthy living through strong partnerships with local, national, and international organizations.

INDEX

Pediatric Environmental Health Specialty
  Units, 2, 5, 16, 23, 46, 65, 66
percentile, 12
personal responsibility, 34
physical properties, 11, 50
physicians, 75
placenta, 74
platelets, 58
playing, 13
pneumonia, 30
pneumonitis, 13
poison, 28
policy, 69
politics, 44
pollution, 5, 20, 68
polyurethane, 11, 31, 67
pools, 32, 33
population, 12, 37, 42, 43, 75
porous materials, 11
prevention, 4, 7, 14, 19, 37, 38, 42, 69
probability sampling, 12
professionals, 24, 70
profit, 67
project, 42
public awareness, 23, 24
public health, 14, 17, 27, 29, 31, 67, 75
public officials, 70
Puerto Rico, 15
pulmonary edema, 13

Q

query, 15, 25, 46

R

rash, 57, 58, 59, 74
real property, 67
recommendations, 37, 69
redevelopment, 32, 67
registry, vii, 1, 2, 8, 38, 39, 46, 47, 76
regression, 40, 60
regulations, 68
remedial actions, 20

remediation, 11, 14, 33
renovated property, vii, 2
resources, 4, 7, 14, 25, 37, 67, 69, 70, 71
respiratory failure, 30
response, 3, 5, 18, 20, 28, 29
risk, 13, 29, 34, 37, 41, 67, 71
risk factors, 34
risk management, 67
risks, 36, 69
room temperature, vii, 3, 4, 9, 19, 73
rules, 68

S

safety, 25, 43, 71, 76
salts, 73
scent, 59, 60, 61
school, 5, 6, 9, 10, 11, 15, 17, 18, 19, 20, 21,
  23, 24, 25, 26, 27, 30, 31, 33, 35, 36, 37,
  38, 39, 40, 41, 42, 44, 48, 50, 51, 53, 57,
  58, 59, 60, 61, 67, 68, 69, 70, 71
science, 6, 9, 11, 25, 30, 35, 37, 38, 47, 49,
  59
search terms, 16
sensation, 28, 58
sex, 5, 23
shellfish, 74
shortness of breath, 59
siblings, 58
signs, 22
silvery liquid, vii, 3, 4, 9
skin, 10, 11, 13, 28, 29, 58, 73, 74
Small Business Liability Relief and
  Brownfields Revitalization Act, 67
software, 20
specialists, 22
species, 12
speech, 60
sphygmomanometer, 28, 33, 43, 48, 49
staff members, 32
stomach, 57
storage, 5, 17, 31, 68
sulfur, 73
Superfund, 1, 16, 25, 46
surface area, 13